# A Clinical Guide To Periodontology

Richard M Palmer,* BDS, PhD, FDS RCS
Peter D Floyd,*† BDS, MSc

*Department of Periodontology and Preventive Dentistry,
UMDS Guy's and St Thomas's Hospitals, London
and †4 Queen Anne Street, London

*Foreword by*

William Becker, DDS, MSD
*Assistant Clinical Professor in Periodontology, University of
Southern California School of Dentistry, Los Angeles, California
and Associate Professor in Periodontology, University of
Texas School of Dentistry, Houston Texas, USA*

1996

Published by the British Dental Association
64 Wimpole Street, London W1M 8AL

Based on articles printed in the British Dental Journal

ISBN 0 904588 48 3

Printed and bound by Craft Print, Singapore

# A Clinical Guide To Periodontology

# Foreword

This well written and beautifully illustrated basic periodontal textbook will serve as a wonderful guide and resource for dental hygienists and dental students wishing to improve their understanding of contemporary periodontics. It can also be of value for dentists wishing to implement periodontal therapy into their practices. The book is a clinical guide covering the basic aspects of periodontal therapy. It offers the reader easy to understand chapters on the most important aspects of treatment without the need to peruse through endless chapters on the basic sciences. The chapter on the essentials of the periodontal examination is clearly written and well illustrated. Comprehension of this chapter will allow the reader to perform a thorough periodontal examination and determine a periodontal diagnosis on the basis of clinical findings. The non-surgical and surgical chapters provide beautifully documented examples of results which can be achieved with various modalities of periodontal therapy. The chapter on dental implants compliments the book and offers viable alternatives for replacement of missing teeth. This book is a must for students or practitioners interested in expanding their understanding of periodontal therapy.

*William Becker*
*Tucson, Arizona*
*1996*

# Preface

This book has been written primarily for general dental practitioners, dental students and dental hygienists. We also hope that postgraduate students will find this to be a useful initial primer. Our aim was to write a concise and straightforward account of periodontal diagnosis and treatment, with an emphasis on the practical application. It is therefore based upon our clinical experience, personal interpretation of the periodontal scientific literature and ideas formulated over many years of postgraduate lecturing.

*RMP*
*PJF*
*London, 1996*

# Acknowledgements

Special thanks to Leslie Smillie for his immense work in designing the layout, copy editing and keeping us on track in the production of this book. We also wish to thank Mike Grace and Tim Newton for their help with chapter 10, James Dewe Mathews for the restorative dentistry shown in chapter 9 and Pauline Floyd for reading and correcting the manuscript.

# Contents

# 1 Periodontal examination and screening

This chapter covers:
1 The BSP/CPITN screening method
2 Periodontal examination
   a. visual examination
   b. periodontal charting
   c. radiographic examination

The majority of adult patients attending a general practice will have suffered from some form of periodontal disease. The clinical features are obvious in the majority of patients, despite many being unaware of their problem. Recognition of more subtle forms of disease requires an increased level of awareness by the clinician. It has been estimated that only about 20% have severe enough disease to result in significant tooth loss, occurring most often in middle to old age. Ideally these individuals should be identified and offered treatment as a priority, preferably at an early stage in the disease process.

It has been shown that initial periodontal attachment loss can be detected in a small proportion of young people in their late teens. Whether they subsequently prove to be the susceptible group identified in older age groups has yet to be established. There are unfortunately no reliable indicators to identify susceptible individuals prior to periodontal breakdown.

Complete periodontal charting of all probing depths in all patients is clearly impractical and unnecessary to accomplish this. A simple method of screening is advocated to facilitate rapid and easy identification of those patients who require treatment and careful monitoring. This is based upon the CPITN system and the modifications proposed by the British Society of Periodontology.

## BSP/CPITN screening

The dentition is divided into sextants (molar/premolar and canine/incisor) and examination carried out with a WHO periodontal probe which has a spherical ended tip (diameter 0.5 mm) and a coloured band extending from 3.5 mm to 5.5 mm. A probing force of approximately 20–25 g is recommended. The probe is gently inserted into the gingival crevice at a minimum of six points on each tooth (mesiobuccal, midbuccal, distobuccal and the corresponding points lingually) or preferably by 'walking' the probe around the tooth to explore the total extent of any pocketing.

For each sextant only the highest score is recorded. A sextant with only one tooth is recorded as missing and the tooth score included in the adjacent sextant. A simple box chart is used to record the scores.

Code 4  Coloured band of the probe disappears into a pocket indicating a probing depth of at least 6 mm.

Code 3  Coloured band of the probe remains partly visible in the deepest pocket of the sextant.

Code 2  Coloured band of the probe remains completely visible in the deepest pocket of the sextant but the presence of calculus or a defective restoration margin is detected supra or subgingivally.

Code 1  Coloured band of the probe remains completely visible in the deepest pocket in the sextant but there is bleeding.

Code 0  Healthy gingival tissue with no bleeding after probing.

Code *  Denotes two special features, either the presence of a furcation involvement or where recession plus the probing depth totals 7 mm or more.

Figure 1 illustrates the different codes. This is a screening system and is not intended to be used for monitoring purposes during treatment or for

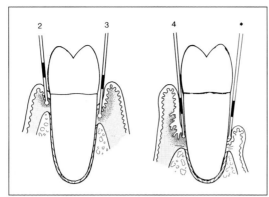

**Fig. 1** Diagrammatic representation of BSP/CPITN screening system illustrating the different codes.

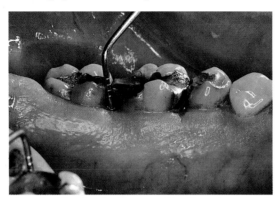

**Fig. 2** Probing depth of 5 mm at distolingual aspect of lower first molar in the presence of healthy, stippled marginal tissue.

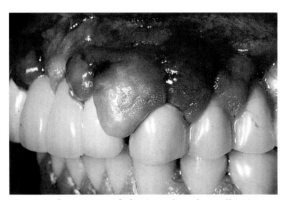

**Fig. 3** Enlargement of the interdental papillae in a patient taking phenytoin. Decementation of an abutment crown on the canine may have further exacerbated the condition.

treatment planning of complex cases. Therefore, those subjects who score 4 or * in any sextant should have a full periodontal chart performed for that sextant (see Periodontal charting on pages 3–4).

## Visual examination

The gingiva is normally pale pink with a fairly noticeable change at the mucogingival junction where the mucosa is redder and blood vessels are visible. Thick healthy marginal tissue may conceal deep seated lesions (fig. 2) which would remain undiagnosed without probing.

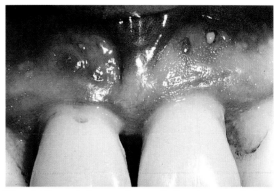

**Fig. 4** Gross inflammation and detachment of the gingiva. Multiple discharging sinuses are present. Loss of stippling is described as one of the early signs of inflammatory changes in the gingiva but, as illustrated here, may persist with severe inflammation and destruction, yet be absent in other individuals with healthy tissue.

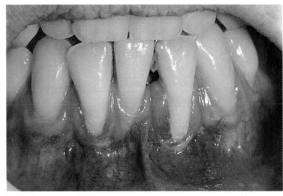

**Fig. 5** Variable degrees of recession on the lower incisors. There is a moderate inflammatory change and the mucogingival junction is close to the gingival margin at the lateral incisors.

Swelling is one of the cardinal signs of inflammation but will differ in consistency and appearance between individuals. Vascular changes occurring in the acute phase of inflammation give rise to oedema and redness. These changes may be exacerbated by such factors as hormonal changes in pregnancy. Fibrotic changes on the other hand are a hallmark of chronic inflammation. More dramatic fibrous enlargement is commonly seen in patients taking phenytoin, cyclosporin and calcium channel blockers such as nifedipine (fig. 3).

The most common complaint in patients with periodontal problems is bleeding, although too often this is accepted as normal. Spontaneous bleeding or the presence of a noticeable purulent exudate occurs in severe disease and may be elicited following periodontal probing or with pressure applied to the gingival tissue (fig. 4).

Gingival recession is a common cause for concern, and is only clinically manifested once the cement enamel junction has become exposed (fig. 5). The receded gingival margin may have all features of gingival health or show inflammation and pocketing. The presence of dark subgingival calculus on the root surface in a supragingival location is proof that prior pocketing existed and that the recession is a result of plaque induced inflammation. Recession associated with excessive toothbrushing is often accompanied by cervical abrasion.

## Periodontal charting

### Probing depths

Conventionally, probing depths are recorded at six points around each tooth, mesial, mid and distal from both the buccal and lingual aspects. At each aspect the examiner should search for the deepest site. Probing depths can be recorded in grids or on pictorial charts, which have the advantage of being able to record other pertinent anatomical facts and help when explaining the clinical situation to the patient (fig. 6). It should be remembered however, that probing depths

> Factors affecting probing
> Force applied
> Probe tip diameter and profile
> Inflammatory status of tissue
> Position of gingival margin
> Presence of subgingival calculus
> Access and crown morphology
> Patient comfort and tolerance

are an approximation of the actual pocket depth and will be influenced by many factors. For the same probing force a probe of a given tip diameter will penetrate further into inflamed tissue than healthy tissue. A decrease in inflammation and the consequent improvement of tissue resistance will result in decreased probe penetration and an apparent gain in attachment. This will be dealt with in more detail in the third article of this series dealing with tissue responses to treatment.

### Furcations

Molar teeth require special consideration because the conventional six-point chart is much less representative of the pattern of disease around multirooted teeth. The estimation of the degree

> Furcation grading
> I   less than 3 mm horizontal probing
> II  greater than 3 mm but not through
> III through and through involvement

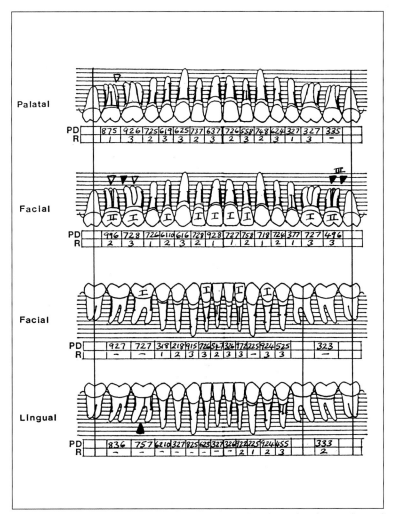

**Fig. 6** Anatomical chart of teeth with numerical and graphical recording of probing depth (PD) and recession (R). Mobilities are recorded in Roman numerals on the crowns. Furcations are recorded in relation to the mesial, distal and buccal aspects of the maxillary teeth as open (grade I) or closed (grade II) triangles. A note is made of any grade III communications.

of destruction within the furcation is difficult but necessary to establish a detailed picture of the remaining support. Furcations can be graded on how far a probe can pass horizontally between the roots but this gives no indication of the vertical destruction on the inner aspects of the furcation. Each furcation entrance is evaluated individually but where roots are close together or the furcation entrance is deeply located, this may be very difficult — even with purpose designed furcation probes. Radiographic examination will help, as will a more thorough evaluation during initial treatment or at the time of surgery.

The furcation grades can be recorded on the chart (fig. 6), where grade 1 is depicted as an open triangle and grade 2 as a filled triangle.

### Recession

It is essential to record the degree of recession as it contributes to the measure of attachment loss (probing depth + recession; fig. 7). Normal clini-

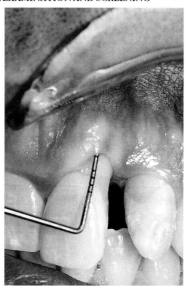

**Fig. 7** Probe in pocket recording a PD of 5 mm and recession of 3 mm giving an attachment loss of 8 mm from the cement–enamel junction.

cal practice rarely records a more coronal position of the gingival margin as with gingival overgrowth. This is also an important feature as it would lead to an overestimation of the degree of destruction caused by an element of false pocketing.

### Mobility

Mobility is usually graded on a 0–3 basis but it remains very subjective. It is normally assessed by applying pressure from the buccal and lingual aspects of the crown using two hand instruments. All teeth have a normal degree of mobility which may only be clinically detectable on teeth with small roots such as lower incisors. Increased mobility occurs with changes resulting from inflammation and increased forces.

Degrees of mobility
0  no detectable movement classically < 0.2 mm
1  horizontal mobility > 0.2 and < 0.5 mm
2  movement 0.5-1 mm
3  > 1 mm or vertical displacement

Factors affecting mobility
Marginal inflammation
Loss of attachment
Widening of periodontal ligament due to increased forces
Loss of apical attachment due to endodontic lesions or root resorption
Unfavourable root morphology, eg short tapering root forms

### Occlusion

The role of occlusion in periodontics is hotly debated. There are a number of circumstances where evaluation of the occlusion, lip competence and parafunctional habits is essential.

When to evaluate the occlusion
Migration of one or a few teeth
Overeruption
Increasing mobility or patient complaining of mobility
Direct tooth to gingival contact as in Class II div 2 incisor relationship
Tooth wear
TMJ symptoms
Treatment plans involving complex restorative work

### Restorative status

An assessment of the restorative and endodontic status of the dentition is obviously vital in reaching a treatment plan and prognosis. Restoration

Restorative factors
Existing restoration
Restorations extending subgingivally and onto root surfaces
Poor quality restoration margins
Caries and recurrent caries
Root caries
Endodontic status
Removable prostheses
Fixed prostheses
Aesthetics

margins extending sub-gingivally, especially if they are poor quality, will directly affect the periodontal tissues by enhancing plaque retention in the most crucial zone (fig. 8).

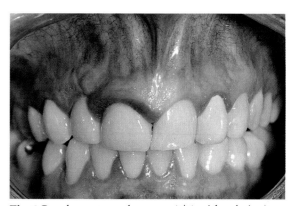

**Fig. 8** Poorly contoured crowns (1|2) with subgingival extension, overhanging margins and poorly contoured embrasure spaces. Increased plaque retention has resulted in severe gingival inflammation.

## Radiographic examination

Routine bitewings in general practice offer a good opportunity to screen patients for periodontal destruction. They should produce minimum distortion even with a short cone. In adults a distance of 2 mm from the cement-enamel junction to interdental bone crest should be considered the normal value. Therefore the bone crest should be visible in both upper and lower jaws, even in early to moderate disease. The bitewing film may also be turned vertically (fig. 9) in order to image the bone crest in more advanced disease. This type of film also has the advantage of being fairly reproducible for long term monitoring in practice.

Periapical films are required for proper assessment of root morphology and length. Those taken with a bisecting angle technique (often with the film bent) are of very limited value because of distortion (fig. 10). The use of a long cone and film holders which facilitate paralleling of tooth and film are recommended (eg Rinn holders).

New generation panoramic tomograms offer a good general evaluation of the teeth and supporting bone and give fairly standard magnification values. However, further development will be required before they can match the quality of images obtainable from intraoral radiographs, particularly in the anterior region which suffers most from distortion and superimposition.

## Conclusion

Many dental practitioners are now using periodontal screening systems during routine dental examinations, and some patients will require more detailed and specific examination. Most patients are unaware of existing periodontal disease and the advantages of early detection are obvious. Overleaf (page 6) is a blank anatomical chart which readers are invited to copy for their own personal use. A blank plaque and bleeding score chart can be found at the end of chapter 2 (page 10).

Subsequent chapters will describe the relatively simple management of early to moderate periodontitis in contrast to complex treatment required in advanced disease.

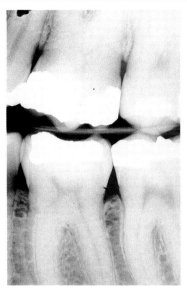

**Fig. 9** Vertical bitewing film showing normal cement–enamel junction to bone crest distance of about 2 mm. The furcations are usually also visible in this type of film.

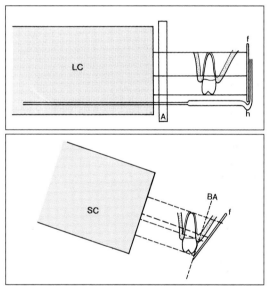

**Fig. 10** Diagram to illustrate difference between longcone paralleling technique (a) and bisecting angle technique (b) in terms of distortion and superimposition of images in the latter.

NAME _____     Date _____

Palatal

PD
R

Facial

PD
R

Facial

PD
R

Lingual

PD
R

Notes

# 2 Periodontal diagnosis and prognosis

**This chapter covers:**
1 Diagnosis
2 Disease progression
3 Risk factors
4 Prognosis

## Diagnosis

The most common periodontal diagnoses to be made are chronic gingivitis and periodontitis. Periodontitis simply means inflammation of the periodontium but is usually interpreted as a destructive chronic inflammatory condition caused by the accumulation of bacterial plaque. However, the term is also applicable to inflammation of the periodontal ligament following trauma or endodontic problems, when it is more accurately described as apical periodontitis. It is accepted that gingivitis is a precursor of periodontitis but that not all gingivitis progresses to periodontitis. A diagnosis of periodontitis means that there has been loss of attachment ie apical migration of the epithelial attachment onto the root surface caused by plaque-induced inflammation.

The differentiation is especially important in young individuals and is most difficult to make in the early transitional stages. In these cases it is necessary to evaluate whether the probe tip at the base of the crevice/pocket is contacting enamel or root surface and to consider the interproximal bone levels on radiographs. Simple features such as whether any subgingival calculus visible on radiographs is located on root or enamel give vital information.

In contrast, gingival recession caused by toothbrush trauma results in visible root surface and loss of attachment. This should not be considered to be periodontitis even in the presence of gingival inflammation. It is a separate and distinct diagnostic entity, requiring different management (which is discussed in chapter 6).

The diagnosis of periodontitis encompasses a wide range of disease entities, some of which fall neatly into specific categories whilst others may be less definable. The commonly recognised diagnostic entities are listed here. However, this series intends to deal only with those which are a major problem in general practice, that is chronic adult periodontitis and gingivitis.

It is useful to subdivide adult periodontitis into severity categories and whether the disease is localised to a few teeth or generalised. Severity can be based upon the amount of bone loss, for instance:

- Early: up to 1/3 bone loss
- Moderate: up to 1/2 bone loss
- Advanced: over 1/2 bone loss and/or involvement of furcations.

Application of these qualifying terms to the diagnosis allows a better description of the disease entity eg 'generalised moderate adult periodontitis' or 'localised advanced periodontitis'.

It is also helpful to categorise pocket probing depths:

- 1–3 mm: normal values
- 4–6 mm: moderate pockets
- 7 mm and over: deep pockets.

The percentage of deep pockets in a patient can be interpreted as a risk factor for disease progression. The distribution of deep pockets when related to tooth anatomy and degree of

Simplified diagnostic categories
**Gingivitis**
Chronic
Hyperplastic
Acute necrotising ulcerative (ANUG)
Acute herpetic
**Periodontitis**
Adult
HIV related
ANUG
**Early onset periodontitis**
Prepubertal
Juvenile
Rapidly progressive

inflammation will have an important influence on decision making in treatment planning and assignment of prognosis.

## Disease progression

The concept of untreated periodontitis progressing slowly and inexorably has been challenged over the last decade. As with many chronic inflammatory conditions it is likely that periodontitis undergoes periods of activity and relative quiescence. Routine clinical probing measurements and radiographs are unable to detect small increments of change. It has been suggested that probing attachment level changes of 2 mm and over are required for the clinician to be more certain of progression, although many such changes are apparently measurement error.

It should be appreciated that monitoring of probing depth alone will often fail to detect disease progression because apical movement of the gingival margin may accompany attachment loss at the depth of the pocket. Sophisticated radiographic techniques including digitised subtraction radiography can detect small changes in crestal height and density provided that the series of radiographs are strictly comparable.

There has also been considerable development of diagnostic test kits (some of which are commercially available) to detect or predict disease progression. In general, they rely upon sampling individual tooth sites which are chosen as either representative of the overall periodontal status or the sites most likely to deteriorate. They are based upon detection of either bacterial species associated with periodontitis (eg *Porphyromonas gingivalis*, *Actinobacillus actinomycetemcomitans*) or components of inflammation (eg neutrophil enzymes, prostaglandins, tissue breakdown products). There is a problem of validating tests against an acceptable 'gold standard' which at the present time has to be clinical measurement with all its attendant inaccuracies.

Currently, the specificity and sensitivity of these tests are not good enough to recommend their use in everyday practice. However, it has been shown that a number of clinical situations are more likely to be associated with disease progression.

Local risk factors for disease
progression
Molar teeth
Maxillary premolars
Proximal surfaces
Advanced attachment loss
A large number of deep pockets

## General risk factors

Risk factors normally apply to the individual and are for the most part difficult to measure, with the exception of age. Moreover, it is impossible to alter or modify the majority of them.

General risk factors
Age
Genetics
  Immunity
  Tooth anatomy
Familial
  bacterial transmission
Stress
Systemic conditions
  eg diabetes
Drugs
  Cytotoxic/immunosuppressive
  Drugs associated with gingival
    overgrowth
Smoking

Tobacco smoking is now a well established risk factor in periodontitis, and one of the few that is possible to modify or eliminate. It has been shown to significantly increase attachment loss and bone loss, whilst reducing bleeding on probing, one of the most obvious signs of inflammation. It also impairs healing following both non-surgical and surgical treatment.

## Prognosis

Periodontal prognosis has been traditionally determined by factors listed below, in particular the severity of disease, age, and subsequently the patients ability and willingness to carry out proper daily plaque removal. A prognosis (eg

Factors affecting prognosis
Age
Clinical factors
  Probing depth
  Loss of attachment
  Furcation involvement
  Restorative/Endodontic
Radiographic factors
  Root length
  Root shape
  Furcation morphology
  Bone height
Aetiological factors
  Plaque
  Calculus
Patient motivation and ability to
  carry out proper plaque control
Operator skill and knowledge
Availability of treatment
  techniques

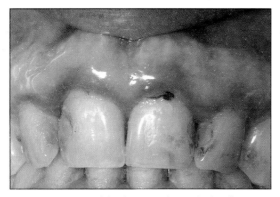

**Fig. 1** A 70-year-old subject with marked inflammation of the marginal gingiva but no loss of attachment ie gingivitis in a highly resistant subject.

good, questionable, hopeless) is often applied to individual teeth as an aid to establishing a treatment plan. However, the first decision often faced by the clinician is whether any teeth should be extracted at an early stage in treatment. Early extraction of teeth considered to be 'hopeless' for periodontal reasons include:

- progression of disease to the point where there is insufficient periodontal ligament support remaining
- the pattern of disease combined with complex/unfavourable root anatomy is such that the tooth is considered to be untreatable.

Formulation of a subsequent definitive treatment plan may indicate further extractions for strategic reasons.

It is also tempting to apply an overall prognosis to the patient's dentition based upon the subjects so-called susceptibility to periodontitis. It is easy to categorise a young patient (say under 35) with moderate or severe disease as being highly susceptible. Likewise it is easy to recognise that an elderly person with gingivitis is resistant (fig. 1). Some clinicians advocate making a judgement based upon the degree of destruction and the amount of plaque and calculus present. This is far more difficult than it would first appear because once a patient has an established periodontitis it provides an ideal environment for increased plaque growth, retention and calcification. The presence of large amounts of plaque and calculus however, may be more helpful in predicting a dramatic response in the tissues following its removal (fig. 2).

## Conclusion

Having established the diagnosis and prognosis an initial treatment plan should be determined together with definitive treatment options for presentation to the patient. The treatment plan

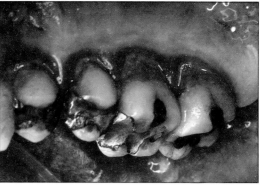

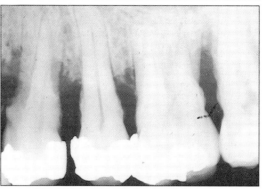

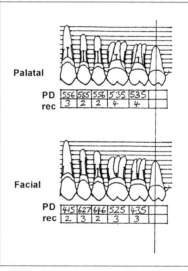

**Fig. 2** A 50-year-old patient with generalised moderate to advanced adult periodontitis. (a) Clinical photograph of palatal view of maxillary posterior teeth showing very inflamed marginal tissue, recession and accumulation of plaque and calculus (previously subgingival). (b) Radiograph showing moderate to advanced bone loss, huge deposits of subgingival calculus and overhanging restoration margins. (c) Clinical charting showing moderate probing depths, recession, furcation involvements and mobilities.

should aim to produce a healthy and functional dentition which is aesthetically acceptable to the patient and within their physical and financial limits.

**NAME**_____

**Plaque Score**_____   **Date**_____

| 8 | 7 | 6 | 5 | 4 | 3 | 2 | 1 | 1 | 2 | 3 | 4 | 5 | 6 | 7 | 8 |
|---|---|---|---|---|---|---|---|---|---|---|---|---|---|---|---|

**Bleeding Score**_____   **Date**_____

| 8 | 7 | 6 | 5 | 4 | 3 | 2 | 1 | 1 | 2 | 3 | 4 | 5 | 6 | 7 | 8 |
|---|---|---|---|---|---|---|---|---|---|---|---|---|---|---|---|

**Plaque Score**_____   **Date**_____

| 8 | 7 | 6 | 5 | 4 | 3 | 2 | 1 | 1 | 2 | 3 | 4 | 5 | 6 | 7 | 8 |
|---|---|---|---|---|---|---|---|---|---|---|---|---|---|---|---|

**Bleeding Score**_____   **Date**_____

| 8 | 7 | 6 | 5 | 4 | 3 | 2 | 1 | 1 | 2 | 3 | 4 | 5 | 6 | 7 | 8 |
|---|---|---|---|---|---|---|---|---|---|---|---|---|---|---|---|

# 3 Non-surgical treatment and maintenance

**This chapter covers:**
1 Supragingival plaque control
2 Subgingival plaque control
3 Role of antimicrobials
4 Maintenance
5 Operator guidelines

The major aetiological agent in chronic periodontitis is bacterial plaque and treatment should be directed at its removal and preventing its re-establishment. Undoubtedly host factors, particularly genetic predisposition, play a major part in disease susceptibility, but they are for the most part not amenable to alteration. An obvious exception to this is tobacco smoking which has quite far reaching effects on inflammation and healing potential. The clinician is however able to eliminate or reduce many of the factors which retain plaque, potentiate its growth and re-establishment or hinder its removal by the patient.

In the initial phase of treatment the role of the patient and clinician should be clearly delineated. The patient should be responsible for the removal of accessible supragingival plaque. These principles apply equally to maintenance care treatment. The patient should be given:
1. A clear explanation of the problem.
2. A treatment plan and the part they play in it.
3. The long term care requirements.
4. An estimate of the time and cost involved.

## Supragingival plaque control

### The patient

Regardless of the level of disease the patient's role in plaque control could be considered as conceptually simple — once daily total removal of supragingival plaque. This goal is rarely achieved, may be unrealistic, and is of less importance in those subjects of lower susceptibility. However, without this aim, particularly in patients of high susceptibility, treatment loses direction and predictability. Motivation of a patient to comply with this aim is a major difficulty in treatment and a number of factors should be considered.

On a practical clinical basis the patient is instructed in mechanical methods of plaque control taking into account physical difficulties and the size and shape of embrasure spaces (table below). Commonly encountered misconceptions/mistakes include:

1. Use of the roll brushing technique in patients with established disease in the belief that it will produce less trauma to the tissue and reduced propensity to recession. Gingival shrinkage is an unavoidable and desirable response to plaque removal indicating a reduction in the

Motivating factors
1. The problem must be important to them
2. They must believe they are susceptible
3. They should believe that treatment is possible and beneficial to them
4. They should understand how to improve the situation
5. They should have the physical skills
6. They need cues to action

Mechanical oral hygiene aids

| Application | Aid/method |
|---|---|
| 1. General brushing | Medium headed nylon toothbrush with miniscrub or bass technique |
| 2. Interproximal surfaces | |
|   2.1 Minimal/no destruction | Floss |
|   2.2 Early destruction | Floss or wooden sticks |
|   2.3 Moderate/severe destruction | Increasing sizes of bottle brushes to cope with larger spaces and root concavities |
| 3. Surfaces adjacent to edentulous spaces, large interproximal spaces and awkward areas. | Single tufted brush |
| 4. Bridge pontics | Superfloss, Floss and threader, bottle brushes |

amount of gingival inflammation. In reality the roll technique is particularly ineffective in removing plaque at a swollen dentogingival junction.

2. Use of floss to clean proximal surfaces which are concave.

3. That antibacterial mouthwashes will significantly reduce established plaque and therefore show a treatment effect on established disease. The place of adjunctive chemical plaque control is discussed later in this chapter (page 15).

4. That scaling is more important than the patient's plaque control in the early stages of treatment.

It must be established in the patient's mind that their efforts in daily plaque control are the single most important factor in determining long term prognosis. Feedback to the patient of their own performance is a good motivator. This is most readily accomplished by demonstrating reduction in the amount of residual supragingival plaque at successive visits. This is best achieved by plaque scoring after disclosing (fig. 1) followed by instruction in how to remove the residual plaque. Disclosed plaque is scored and a record kept. Additional instruction is then given to enable the patient to remove the plaque — which they should accomplish whilst in the chair.

*The clinician*

In addition to instruction and monitoring the patients plaque control, the clinician should reduce or remove factors which hinder the patients efforts to remove plaque close to, or beneath, the gingival margin.

> Factors which hinder patients plaque control or retain plaque
> 1. Calculus
> 2. Poor restoration margins
> 3. Over-contoured restorations and lack of embrasure space
> 4. Removable partial dentures/ appliances particularly those that cover large areas of gingival margin.

Supragingival calculus is simple to remove with push scalers, sickle scalers and/or ultrasonic scalers. The technical aspects of this are dealt with on pages 17 and 18. Prevention of the reformation of supragingival calculus is much more difficult in some individuals than others. A common mistake made by many clinicians is to place undue importance on supragingival calculus and to spend the majority of their time on its removal rather than attending to the more important subgingival plaque and calculus.

Restoration margins close to, or extending beneath, the gingival margin are major plaque retentive factors when overhangs are present. Poorly condensed amalgam overhangs can often be dealt with by hand instruments and ultrasonic scalers. However rotary instruments using coarse and fine finishing burs are needed for harder restorative materials (fig. 2). Gradual shrinkage of the inflamed gingival margins makes access to them easier.

*Assessment*

An assessment of the patients ability to perform a good standard of oral hygiene is relatively easy and is based upon their plaque scores. There should also be a concomitant reduction in marginal inflammation but this will also depend upon the clinician's success with correction of supragingival factors and more importantly subgingival plaque, which is dealt with in the next section.

## Subgingival plaque control

*The patient*

It is unrealistic to expect the patient to remove plaque from the subgingival area with exception of the first millimetre or so of the crevice. It is also a common misconception that mouthwashes flow beneath the gingival margin.

Their action is supragingival unless direct irrigation into the pockets with a cannula is performed.

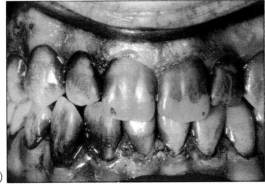

(a)

(b)

**Fig. 1** (a) Upper incisor teeth with disclosed plaque. The blue staining plaque is more mature and is scored on the basis of being present or absent at the dentogingival junction on any of the four cervical teeth surfaces — mesial, distal, buccal, lingual. (b) The plaque score chart corresponding to the anterior region shown in (a). The plaque score for whole mouth is a simple calculation and equals the number of positive surfaces divided by the number of teeth × 4, × 100.

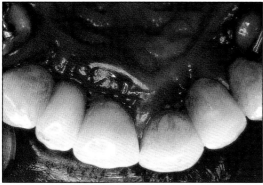

(a)

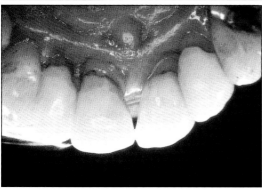

(b)

**Fig. 2** (a) Palatal view of crowned upper incisor teeth with overcontoured PJCs which have large overhangs. The palatal tissue is very inflamed. (b) Resolution of inflammation following non-surgical treatment and recontouring of restorations with high speed finishing burs. Replacement of the crowns is now possible.

## The clinician

Subgingival plaque is an extremely complex mass of bacteria adhering to the root surface, calcifying in some areas to produce hard dark subgingival calculus. It extends into the root surface imperfections and exposed cementum and also has a non-adherent phase within the pocket. Removal of all these noxious elements is very difficult and impossible to determine. Terminology is similarly confusing. Root planing implies removal of cementum (and possibly dentine) exposed within the pocket to maximise the chance of removing all components of the subgingival plaque. If using hand instruments the clinician uses the smoothness of the root surface as the criterion for completion. Subgingival scaling is the removal of deposits of subgingival calculus detected by touch. In reality the procedures are similar.

PRACTICAL AND TECHNICAL ASPECTS
The majority of patients undergoing root planing need local anaesthesia. A combination of hand instruments and ultrasonic scalers is recommended to cope with variations in root anatomy, pocket morphology and operator fatigue. In controlled clinical trials equivalent results have been achieved with both forms of instrumentation.

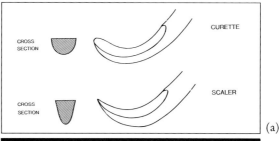

(a)

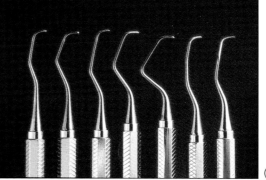

(b)

**Fig. 3** (a) The sickle scaler has a sharp point and triangular cross section compared with the more rounded profile of the curette (reproduced with permission from *The clinical handling of dental materials*, Butterworth-Heinemann, 1994). (b) Gracey curettes. This figure illustrates curettes within the Gracey range. Unlike the universal curette illustrated in (a) they have a cutting edge on one side only. The patterns which prove to be most useful in the majority of cases are: 1/2 anterior teeth, 7/8 premolar teeth — buccal and lingual surface of molar teeth, 11/12 mesial surfaces of molar teeth, 13/14 distal surfaces of molar teeth.

Sickle scalers, such as MacFarlane 4/5, while being the instrument of choice for supragingival scaling, are not suitable for subgingival use. Curettes which have a rounded end (fig. 3a) are recommended. A small bladed double ended universal curette such as the Barnhardt 5/6 or Columbia 4L/4R will tackle most root surfaces. However in deep and narrow pockets, specialised instruments such as the Gracey range are preferred (fig. 3b). Periodontal hoes are liked by some clinicians but care needs to be exercised to avoid grooving root surfaces and the flat ends do not conform to concave root surfaces.

Careful instrumentation requires firm grasping of the instrument in a pengrip and using the first/second finger as a rest. Good technique entails wrist movement using the fingers as a fulcrum. This considerably reduces operator fatigue. The cutting action of the instrument relies upon it subtending the correct angle to the root surface. This is illustrated in figure 4.

Ultrasonic instrumentation should be carried out using a fine tip such as the cavitron p10 and plenty of coolant. The tip should be kept in motion and the surface instrumented with vertical and horizontal movements so as to ensure complete coverage of the root surface. The ultrasonic scaler gives less tactile feedback to the

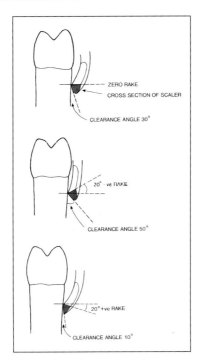

**Fig. 4** Cross section of a curette against a root surface. This illustration shows the variation in angle when the cutting edge is still effective (reproduced with permission from *The clinical handling of dental materials*, Butterworth-Heinemann, 1994).

clinician and therefore evaluating the surface with a hand instrument is important. Whilst the surface should feel smooth and hard it is impossible to determine the completeness of plaque removal. This is based largely upon experience of treating a wide range of cases and thereby establishing the time and effort required to produce a satisfactory clinical response. As a guide, an experienced clinician would allow about 45 minutes to root plane seven teeth with moderately deep pockets. There is a large number of factors which will reduce the effectiveness of subgingival instrumentation and hence the chance of a successful outcome.

Handicaps to successful instrumentation
1. Pocket depth — especially over 6 mm
2. Complex root shapes — especially molar furcations
3. Difficult access — posterior teeth and limited mouth opening
4. Instruments — inappropriate, too large or dull
5. Patient co-operation — discomfort or powerful oral musculature
6. Operator skill

INSTRUMENT SHARPENING

Root planing is impossible with dull instruments. It is relatively easy to keep an instrument sharp by using a sterile oiled stone during the procedure. Renovating a very blunt instrument requires much more effort and often extensive reshaping with a rotary stone. In simple terms the cutting edge of the curette or sickle scaler can be redefined by removing a small quantity of metal from the face of the blade or preferably from the side of the blade (fig. 5). This latter method can be accomplished stroking the in-

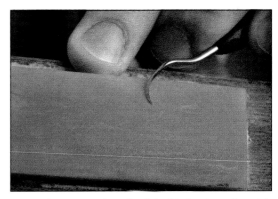

**Fig. 5** Sharpening the side of the blade of a scaler with a flat stone.

strument on a flat stone and is technically less demanding than using a round stone on the blade face.

*Assessment*

Success of non-surgical periodontal treatment is based almost entirely on clinical measurement. In untreated disease the periodontal probe penetrates the base of the pocket into the inflamed connective tissue which offers low resistance (fig. 6). This will also result in bleeding from the depth of the pocket. Bleeding can also be scored in a simple fashion of present or absent, and graphically displayed as a score in exactly the same way as the plaque score (see page 12). Following removal of supra- and subgingival plaque there should be a marked reduction in inflammation. The reduction of the fluid and cellular components of the inflammatory lesion should result in shrinkage producing gingival recession and an increasing proportion of colla-

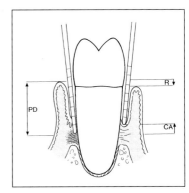

**Fig. 6** Diagrammatic representation of a probe in an untreated pocket (left). The probing depth (6 mm) is measured from the gingival margin, which in this case is about 1 mm coronal to the cement enamel junction. Note the probe enters the inflamed connective tissue at the base of the pocket. The right side represents a favourable response to non-surgical treatment. The probing depth has reduced to 4 mm. The 2 mm reduction is made up of 1 mm gingival shrinkage and 1 mm decreased penetration of the probe at the base of the pocket. This latter improvement is referred to as a gain in clinical attachment.

gen fibres within the gingival connective tissue, which combined with establishment of a long junctional epithelium will produce increased resistance to the passage of the probe tip. Gingival recession is the first change noticed, usually within one week, whereas the change in probe penetration is more gradual taking 4–6 weeks.

The reductions obtained in probing depth as a result of non-surgical periodontal treatment are usually within the range of 1–2 mm which is the width of the black or coloured band on the WHO probe recommended for CPITN scores. Therefore it is possible that a record of code 3 could be scored both before and after treatment. The BSP/CPITN system of screening examination was not designed for and is not suitable for patient monitoring.

Complete resolution of inflammation should be achievable in both gingivitis and early to moderate periodontitis with well performed non-surgical management. This will obviously depend upon coping with the factors given in the panel on page 14 and the individual patient's response to plaque removal. Patients with more overt inflammatory changes and less fibrosis of the gingival tissue respond in a more dramatic fashion with marked shrinkage of the marginal tissue, thereby producing a result which looks as though there has been some surgical excision (fig. 7). A good example of individuals who respond less well are tobacco smokers. In these patients smok-

ing reduces the inflammatory changes and bleeding in untreated disease (while conversely increasing bone and attachment loss) and detrimentally affects the healing response in both non-surgical and surgical treatment.

## Role of antimicrobials

Antimicrobials can be used to supplement or substitute (1) the patient's oral hygiene programme or (2) the clinician's mechanical plaque removal.

### The patient

The most widely used antimicrobial in periodontal treatment is chlorhexidine mouthwash. It is undoubtedly the most effective chemical agent for the control of supragingival plaque and gingivitis. It is particularly useful when the gingival tissues are too sore or fragile to withstand normal cleaning procedures, such as following periodontal surgery.

It is not recommended for indefinite use as this makes it difficult to determine how well the patient is cleaning. The side effects of staining and the affect on taste often limit patient acceptability. Other mouthwashes containing antiseptic agents have some adjunctive benefit but it is unlikely that the currently available prebrushing rinses offer a significant advantage in the treatment of patients with periodontitis.

### The clinician

Mechanical removal of plaque using methods described in this article should result in marked improvements in periodontal health with little need to consider adjunctive antimicrobials. Systemically administered antibiotics such as tetracycline and metronidazole may be indicated in extreme forms of periodontitis such as rapidly progressive periodontitis, but should not be used routinely. Locally administered formulations of these antibiotics are now marketed and have the advantage of minimising systemic absorption whilst maintaining therapeutic levels within the pocket. They show some additional pocket reduction at initially deep sites when used in conjunction with root planing, but the adjunctive effect is relatively small. Locally delivered antimicrobials are occasionally recommended to help maintain sites which prove to be refractory to well delivered treatment. Proof of long term benefit is difficult to establish.

## Maintenance

All patients who have received non-surgical and surgical treatment require maintenance care at varying levels and intervals dependent upon:

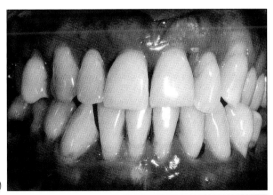
(a)

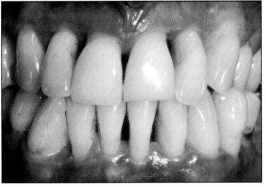
(b)

**Fig. 7** (a) A patient with advanced periodontitis before treatment showing signs of gross inflammation and oedema. (b) The patient showing dramatic reduction in inflammation just 2 weeks following root planing.

1. Initial severity of disease and patient's susceptibility.

2. Degree of difficulty of instrumentation of residual pockets following treatment.

3. Level of patient's supragingival plaque control.

Some of these factors are difficult to quantify and ultimately maintenance schedules may be gradually established over the first year or two following active treatment. Whilst the most commonly quoted maintenance interval is 3-monthly, more susceptible individuals may require 2-monthly intervals and more resistant patients extended to 4- or 6-monthly. In many

### Response to non-surgical treatment

This simplified approach is to give some basic guidelines and should be interpreted with caution. Future treatment decisions are complex and also relate to such factors as disease severity at initial diagnosis, improvement gained with treatment, and complexity of residual problems.

| | Ideal | Satisfactory | Unsatisfactory |
|---|---|---|---|
| **Plaque score** | < 15% | >15% and under 40% dependent upon susceptibility | >40% |
| **Probing depths** | 1 to 3 mm | Most 1–4 mm, few 4–6 mm | many > 4 mm,* some > 6 mm |
| **Furcation involvement** | None | Early Grade I or incipient | Some Grade 1 plus Grade II/III |
| **Bleeding score (*non*-smokers)** | < 10% | > 10 and < 40% dependent upon susceptibility | > 40% |
| **Future treatment options** | Simple maintenance | 1. Surgery if plaque scores are low 2. Maintenance with subgingival removal of plaque from residual pockets and re-evaluation in 1 year | 1. Improve plaque scores and re-treat 2. Extract untreatable teeth 3. Maintain as best as possible |

*The number of probing depths over 4 mm is a risk indicator for disease progression

practices maintenance and most of the non-surgical treatment is delegated to the hygienist. Under these circumstances it is essential for the clinician who is responsible for the patient to ensure that the appropriate level and frequency of treatment is delivered. Annual re-evaluations are important in this regard when decisions may have to be made whether to change the maintenance schedule, increase the level of care or re-treat specific sites.

Another common error in clinical management is simply to place patients into a 3-monthly maintenance schedule without delivering the appropriate level of definitive treatment in the first place. Further difficulties arise when patients exercise their rights and refuse to have hopeless teeth extracted. Under these circumstances it is normally incumbent on the clinician to at least deliver a level of care which will

minimise the chance of acute exacerbations or damage to adjacent teeth. However the patient should be fully informed that they are keeping the tooth against the clinician's advice and that the particular tooth is not in any way suitable to be included as a viable unit in a treatment plan, especially those that involve complex restorative dentistry. A typical maintenance appointment would include as necessary:

1. A review of the patient's plaque control (ideally following disclosing and scoring) and reinforcement.

2 . A check on defect probing depths and removal of any subgingival plaque from pockets over 4 mm (particularly those that bleed) and furcation involvements.

3. A supragingival prophylaxis.

## Conclusion

Non-surgical treatment produces some of the most dramatic and significant improvements in periodontal health. The majority of patients in general practice should be completely treated using these simple techniques. Those patients who finish treatment with normal probing depths in the 1–3 mm category and little or no bleeding on probing should be maintainable with supragingival cleaning and little professional intervention.

Others may, despite well performed treatment and maintenance of good supragingival cleaning, have residual pockets which can harbour plaque and require surgical therapy or more professionally administered maintenance care in the form of regular subgingival plaque removal. Some simplified guidelines are given on the left.

## Operator guidelines

Periodontal treatment procedures are time-consuming and adoption of good working practices will considerably reduce fatigue and increase efficiency. The remaining pages in this chapter form a pictorial guide to scaling and root planing. A series of photographs describing the optimum positions for instrumenting various regions of the mouth is followed by a guide on the use of a sickle scaler as an example of a 'universal' instrument. There is then an outline of the types of Gracey curettes, along with a number of examples of where and how they should be used.

In addition, the information in this section applies to the use of ultrasonic scalers, which are often used in combination with hand instruments. The reader should also find this a useful guide to operator/patient positioning for periodontal surgical procedures.

# Positioning of the operator and patient for scaling

This series of photographs (figs 8–12) illustrates suggestions for operating in various regions of the mouth. The position of the operator is described in relation to a clockface where the headrest of the chair is at 12 o'clock.

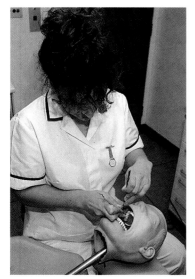

**↑Fig. 8 Upper right buccal**
1. Operator at 10 o'clock. 2. Patient's head turned away slightly. 3. Cheek retracted with mirror. 4. Finger rest on adjacent teeth.

**→Fig. 9 Upper left palatal showing two approaches**
(a) 1. Operator at 10 o'clock. 2. Patient's head turned away slightly. 3. Cheek retracted with mirror. 4. Remote finger rest.
(b) 1. Operator at 9 o'clock. 2. Patient's head turned away slightly. 3. Mirror used to reflect light. 4. Finger rest on adjacent teeth. 5. Palm cupped around patient's chin.

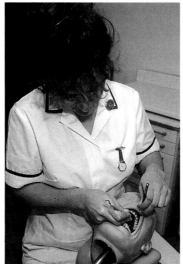

(a)

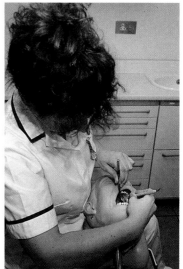

(b)

Fundamental points to bear in mind for efficient and comfortable operating (fig. 10)
1 Operator seated low with thighs parallel to the floor.
2 Operator has upright posture with straight back.
3 Operator at 11 o'clock.
4 Patient reclined so that head is almost within the operator's lap.
5 Patient's head is 'well up' on the head rest.
6 Operator's arms at comfortable level.
7 Instruments stabilised with finger rests.
This allows direct vision to many areas and can be improved by:
1 Rotating patient's head.
2 Reclining headrest to extend patient's neck allows better access to the palate.
The operator should not be contorting but should move the patient into a position which facilitates access.

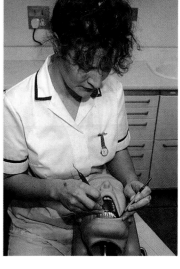

**Fig. 10**

**↓Fig. 11 Lower left lingual**
1. Operator at 10/11 o'clock. 2. Patient's head turned away slightly. 3. Tongue retracted with mirror and light reflected. 4. Finger rest on anterior teeth and instrument grip extended to compensate.

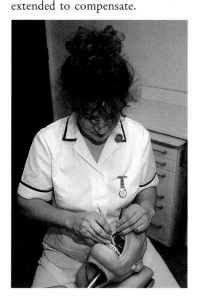

**→Fig. 12 Lower right showing two approaches**
(a) Lingual. 1.Operator at 11 o'clock. 2. Patient's head turned towards operator slightly. 3. Tongue retracted with mirror. 4. Finger rest on adjacent teeth. (b) Buccal. 1. Operator at 7 o'clock. 2. Patient's head straight. 3. Cheek retracted with mirror. 4. Finger rest on anterior teeth.

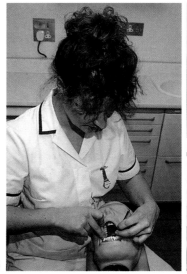

(a)

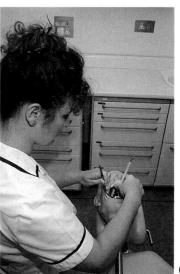

(b)

## Use of a sickle scaler

The operator is seated at 12 o'clock and a finger rest taken close to, but not immediately adjacent to the tooth (fig. 13). The working tip is introduced inter-proximally and applied to the distal surface of 31 (fig. 14). The tip is then moved in a apical direction to below the calculus deposit (fig. 15) prior to the working stroke.

There is a slight difference in angulation required when the mesial surface of 32 is instrumented. This is illustrated in figure 16 (tooth 31 distal) and figure 17 (tooth 32 mesial). The difference in angulation can normally be achieved by movement of the hand (in this instance towards the mid-line) without necessarily moving the finger rest. There are a number of different sickle scalers and universal curettes which are used in a similar manner. Their use is indicated in different areas according to the shank length and angle.

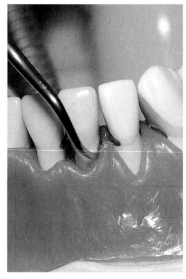

**Fig. 16**

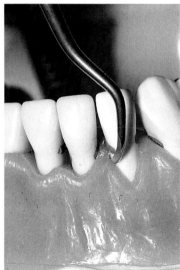

**Fig. 17**

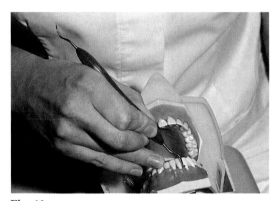

**Fig. 13**

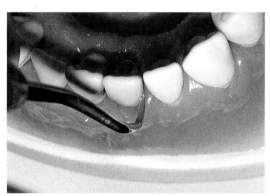

**Fig. 14**

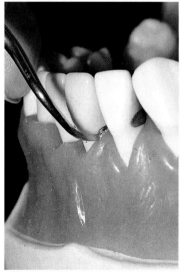

**Fig. 15**

## Gracey pattern curettes

These are a set of specialised curettes (fig. 18) designed for various tooth surfaces made possible by the complex bends in the shanks and the blade design. The blades have only one cutting surface (not two as with universal curettes) such that a negative rake angle is achieved when the terminal shank is parallel with the long axis of the root surface.

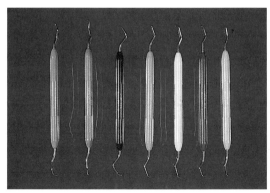

**Fig. 18** Gracey pattern curettes. Left to right: 1/2, 3/4, 5/6, 7/8, 9/10, 11/12, 13/14.

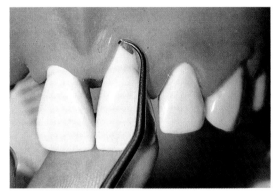

**Fig. 19**

## Gracey curette #1/2: Anterior teeth all surfaces

These figures show the use of the Gracey curette #1/2 for use on anterior teeth. The instrument is held with the terminal shank (ie second portion of shank closest to the blade) roughly parallel to the long axis of the tooth (fig. 20). The finger rest is normally on the same or adjacent tooth (figs 19 and 20). The working tip of the instrument is introduced subgingivally (fig. 21) and kept in gentle contact with the root surface and/or calculus deposit until the base of the pocket is reached. The working stroke is then commenced. The working movement of the instrument is parallel to the axis of the terminal shank.

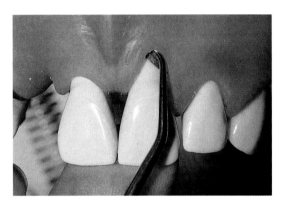

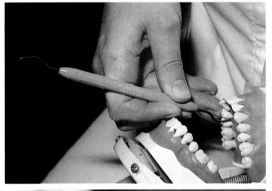

**Fig. 20**

**Fig. 21**

## Gracey pattern curette #7/8:
## Buccal and palatal aspects of premolar/molar teeth

Figure 22 shows (a) Access and finger rest positions for treating the palatal aspects of the upper right premolars. (b) Close up view of the #7/8 on the palatal aspect of the upper right first premolar. Figure 23 shows (a) The #7/8 applied to the buccal aspect of the upper left molars. (b) A close up view of the #7/8 on the buccal aspect of the upper left first molar.

(a)

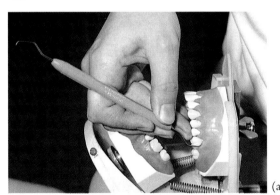

(a)

(b)

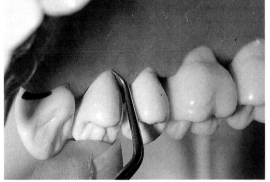

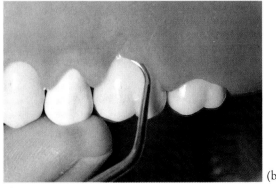

(b)

**Fig. 22**

**Fig. 23**

**19**

## Gracey pattern curette #13/14: Distal surfaces of molar teeth

The terminal shank of the Gracey pattern curette #13/14 is held approximately parallel to the root surface to be instrumented. It is important to remember that root morphology is variable and poor access sometimes makes it difficult to achieve the correct angulation.

Figure 24 shows the finger rest on the anterior teeth with the instrument at the distal aspect of the lower first molar. In figure 25 the #13/14

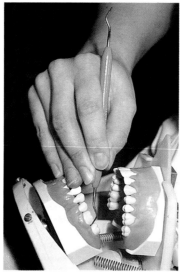

**Fig. 24**

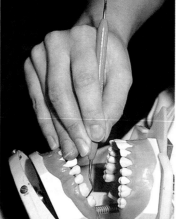

**Fig. 25**

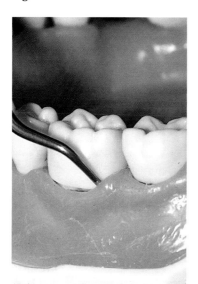

**Fig. 26**

blade is at the distal surface of the lower first molar. The instrument blade has a negative rake angle which in this figure is too great, ie the tip or blade of the instrument is 'closed' against the root surface and the cutting/cleaving action is negated. The terminal shank

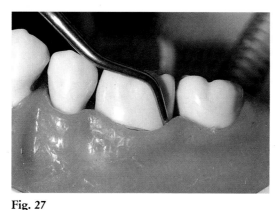

**Fig. 27**

should be parallel with the root surface (see fig. 27). Figure 26 shows the #13/14 introduced into the pocket trying to maintain an effective rake angle, at a site which has quite difficult access. In figure 27the terminal shank is more in line with the long axis of the root surface, producing a more effective rake angle.

## Gracey pattern curette #11/12: Mesial surfaces of molar teeth (and universal application)

The Gracey curette #11/12 is primarily designed for treatment of the mesial aspects of the posterior teeth. In common with some other specialised instruments, it also has a wider application to many other surfaces including the anterior teeth and buccal and lingual of the posterior teeth.

Figure 28 shows (a) Access to the mesial (palatal) aspect of the upper right molar. (b) Close up view showing angle of blade to tooth surface. (c) Close up view showing instrument inserted into pocket maintaining angle of blade to the root surface. The terminal shank of the instrument is parallel with the long axis of the root surface.

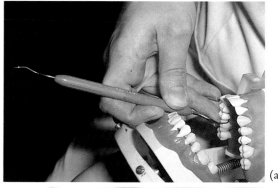

(a)

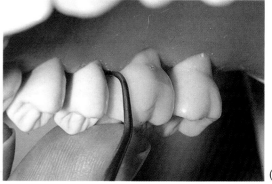

(b)

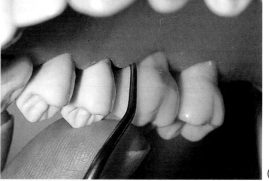

(c)

**Fig. 28**

Figure 29 shows (a) Access to the mesial (buccal) aspect of lower left second molar. (b) Close up view showing angle of blade to tooth surface. (c) Close up view showing instrument inserted into pocket maintaining angle of blade to the root surface.

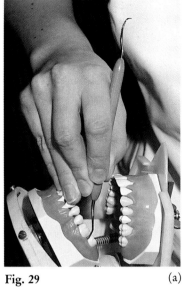 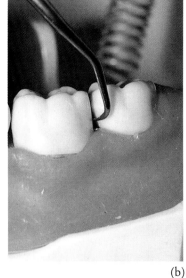 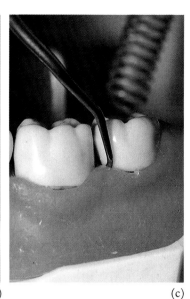

**Fig. 29**         (a)                    (b)                    (c)

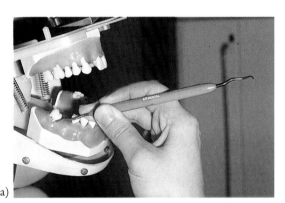

(a)

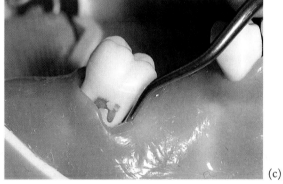

(c)

Figure 30 shows (a) Access to the mesial aspect of a tilted lower right second molar with the operator seated at 7 o'clock. (b) Close up view showing angle of blade to mesial tooth surface demonstrating the rake angle. (c) Close up view showing instrument inserted into pocket maintaining angle of blade to the root surface.

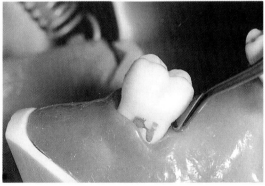

(b)

**Fig. 30**

# 4

# Periodontal surgery

**This chapter covers:**
1 **The indications for surgery**
2 **Surgical methods**
3 **Periodontal flap surgery**
4 **Surgical management of the palate and tuberosity**

The majority of patients with chronic periodontitis suffer from mild to moderate disease and should be treatable with non-surgical methods. Moderate pocketing of 4–6 mm should thereby be reduced in most instances to near normal probing depths (less than or equal to 4 mm) with little or no residual bleeding on probing. Deep pockets, those 7 mm and over, show the most marked reductions in probing depths during non-surgical treatment but are obviously much more likely to result in some degree of persistent pocketing. The consistency of the soft tissues will also have a profound effect on the gingival response during non-surgical treatment, even in pockets of moderate depth. There is much less potential for recession in fibrotic tissues as compared with those tissues which initially showed a marked oedematous/inflammatory component.

## Indications

There are no hard and fast rules governing when periodontal surgery is chosen as a treatment modality, but certain clinical observations increase the likelihood. Periodontal surgery may therefore be required in those patients who on presentation show:

1. Pockets greater than 6 mm.

2. Pockets associated with thick fibrous gingiva.

3. Furcation involvement (to be covered in detail in part 5 of this series).

4. Mucogingival deformities or extensive periodontitis lesions requiring reconstructive or regenerative treatment (see chapter 6).

5. Short clinical crowns where an increase in clinical crown height is required before restorations are constructed (see chapter 7).

It is helpful to consider the aims of periodontal surgery. Previously, one of the major aims of periodontal surgery was the treatment of progressive disease persisting after a phase of non-surgical treatment. The detection of progressive disease is fraught with difficulties and for the most part has relied upon clinical and radiographic changes such as:

1. Bleeding or pus on probing the depths of the pockets.

2. Clinical measures of loss of attachment.

3. Radiographic evidence of bone loss.

Unfortunately all these proposed indicators have major drawbacks. For instance the presence of bleeding or pus are not specific or sensitive enough. Clinical measurements suffer from large errors. The variation in tissue resistance due to the degree of inflammatory infiltrate can result in substantial differences in probing attachment level without a change in the level of connective tissue attachment to the root surface. If detection of 'disease activity' is difficult the prediction of future 'disease activity' is practically impossible. In contrast, the presence of gingival health (which we have defined as normal looking gingivae with no bleeding or discharge in probing depths of 4 mm and below) has proved to be the best predictor of future stability.

Surprisingly, radiographic examination in clinical practice is no more reliable. Although accurate radiographic techniques such as subtraction radiography used by research workers

> **Aims of periodontal surgery**
> 1. Gain access to previously inaccessible root surfaces
> 2. Produce a healthy dentogingival junction that the patient can keep free of plaque
> 3. Predictably reduce probing depths thereby simplifying:
>    3.1 professionally delivered maintenance care
>    3.2 the detection of recurrent inflammation
>    3.3 the detection of progressive periodontal destruction

are available, clinicians find it difficult to produce comparable radiographs. The use of film holders and a long cone paralleling technique overcomes some of these difficulties and is highly recommended and used routinely by the authors.

Most importantly, both the clinician and patient should be aware of the limitations of periodontal surgery.

> Limitations of periodontal surgery
> 1 It will not compensate for the patient's poor plaque control, nor necessarily facilitate plaque control by exposing more root surface area which has more complex anatomy.
> 2 It will not alter the prognosis of untreatable teeth.
> 3 It is unlikely to eradicate complex deformities resulting from disease such as deep grade II and grade III furcations.
> 4 It will not produce miraculous and complete regeneration of all lost periodontal tissues.
> 5 There will normally be an apical shift in the position of the dentogingival junction which may compromise aesthetics to some degree.

## Surgical methods

Conceptually the easiest surgical method is excision, which is exemplified by the gingivectomy. This is a very useful procedure in reducing excess gingival tissue such as that occurring with drug-induced overgrowth (fig. 1). It will not effectively deal with pockets which extend apically to the crestal bone (infrabony pockets) which are very common in moderate to advanced periodontitis. In addition, it should not be used where it will result in total excision of the gingiva. In contrast, periodontal flap surgery is a more flexible approach, in which it is possible to retain keratinised gingiva while treating pockets of any depth and facilitates the positioning of the flap margin at any desired level.

Before considering periodontal surgery the clinician should be satisfied that:

1. The patient has been maintaining a good level of oral hygiene (low plaque scores) and that this is likely to continue.

2. Adequate time and effort have been applied to the non-surgical phase of treatment.

3. The patient is willing to enrol on a suitable maintenance programme within the immediate postoperative period and subsequently.

4. The teeth are technically treatable.

5. The patient is aware of the limitations and is fit to undergo the procedures.

## Periodontal flap surgery

### Preoperative preparation

The clinician should have available a recent probing depth chart and radiographs. All periodontal surgery can be readily accomplished under local anaesthesia. Local anaesthetics containing adrenaline help to reduce bleeding and improve visibility in the operative field. Buccal and palatal infiltrations are given in the maxilla, and block anaesthesia together with some local infiltration in the mandible. It is a good idea to give the patient some analgesics such as ibuprofen or paracetamol before commencing the procedure to give some analgesia as the local anaesthesia wears off postoperatively. Some clinicians also like to give a chlorhexidine mouthwash just before the procedure or immediately afterwards. As in all good surgical practice the procedure should be performed with sterile instruments and gloves using a no-touch technique.

### Periodontal surgical technique

Periodontal flap surgery is described here using a series of clinical photographs and explanatory diagrams (figs 2–11) together with a description

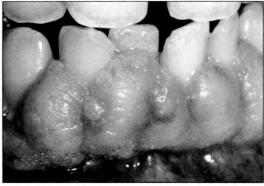
(a)

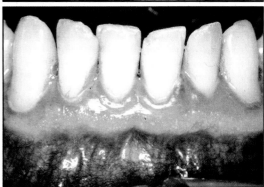
(b)

**Fig. 1** (a) Epanutin-induced gingival overgrowth before treatment. (b) Following gingivectomy and a healing period of 3 months.

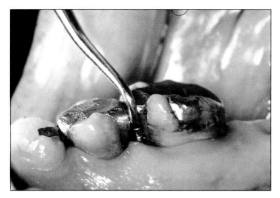

**Fig. 2** Preoperative view of the lingual aspect of lower premolar and molar teeth. A probe is shown recording a depth of 8 mm on the mesial aspect of the first molar. It should be noted that the gingival tissue is free of superficial inflammation and the supragingival plaque control is good.

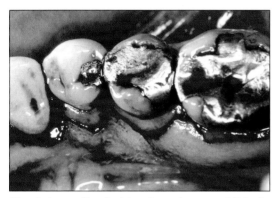

**Fig. 3** An outline incision is made to establish the shape of the flap by cutting into the tissue to a depth of no more than 1 to 2 mm.

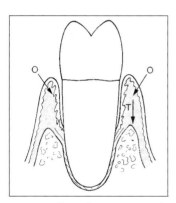

**Fig. 4** Diagram to show the position and angle of the outline incision (O) and subsequent development of this incision (T) extending to the bone crest. The outline incision is made at a convenient angle for the clinician and is normally at about 30 degrees to the long axis of the tooth. The secondary or thinning incision is used to separate a flap of adequate thickness from the soft tissue of the pocket wall and the angle is dictated by the surface contour of the gingiva.

of the important features. A mandibular molar area has been chosen to show some of the complications when dealing with more difficult areas.

Ideally the flap is shaped to match the contours of the teeth at the position it will occupy at the end of the procedure. The incision is

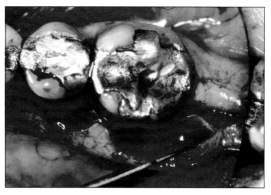

**Fig. 5** Completion of the secondary incision showing its extension into the edentulous space distal to the first molar. In this figure the no. 15 blade is being used with the cutting edge uppermost in a filleting action.

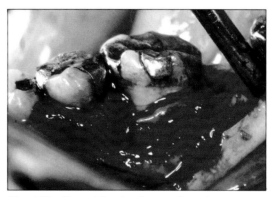

**Fig. 6** The lingual flap has been reflected to expose 2 to 3 mm of bone. The soft tissue of the pocket wall is still attached to the teeth and bone crest.

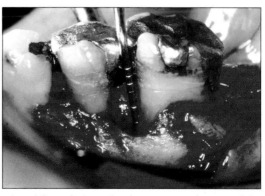

**Fig. 7** The soft tissue has been removed to reveal the root surfaces. There is a deep bone defect on the mesial aspect of the first molar from which soft inflammatory tissue has been removed. The furcation is intact.

normally accomplished with a no. 15 blade but because of the more difficult access on the lingual aspect of the lower molars a no. 12 blade is often used.

The optimal thickness of the flap is about 1.5 to 2 mm and therefore a variable width of soft tissue/pocket lining will be left next to the tooth. In areas where the gingival tissue is very thin the flap will need to conserve the entire thickness of the available soft tissue. It is very

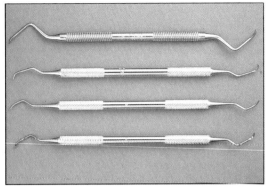

**Fig. 8** Surgical curettes used for removing soft tissue and root planing. At the top is a Prichard curette and below that three Goldman Fox curettes. Occasionally finer instruments such as those used in non-surgical treatment are required to instrument narrow defects. The Gracey range are available in a more rigid pattern and are ideal for this purpose.

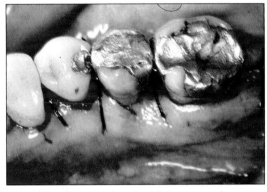

**Fig. 9** The flaps are closed with interrupted sutures.

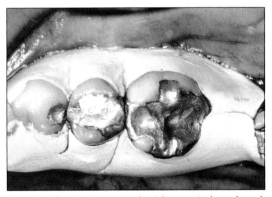

**Fig. 10** The site is covered with a periodontal pack which should remain in place until the patient is seen for suture removal in 1 week.

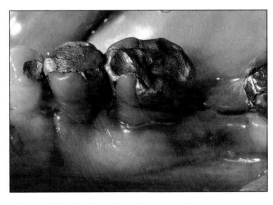

**Fig. 11** The healing site after 1 week.

important to avoid overthinning the flap as this will lead to necrosis, appearing as ulceration, after a few days. The secondary or thinning incision is made with a no. 15 blade using a careful filleting action. The incision is completed to the marginal bone, ideally just on its outer aspect. A periosteal elevator is introduced into the incision and the flap gently reflected to reveal a small amount of marginal bone.

If undue force is required then first consider:

1. The incision may not be complete. This frequently occurs where the bone margin is irregular.

2. The incision may have been carried into a bone defect such as an interdental crater or circumferential gutter.

In either case the incision should be completed to the bone crest to facilitate reflection and avoid tearing the flap.

Both buccal and lingual flaps should be completed and elevated to expose crestal bone before removing the soft tissue of the pocket wall, which may otherwise still be attached to the flaps. The flaps should be carefully protected during the removal of the pocket lining and inflammatory tissue with curettes. Surgical curettes such as the Goldman Fox series are ideal for this purpose as they are larger and stronger than the instruments used for non-surgical treatment. These instruments are then used to plane the root surfaces. Ultrasonic scalers are also very useful for this purpose, particularly as access has been optimised and the irrigant produces a clear washed field for visual inspection.

The minimal reflection of flaps during the procedure helps to reduce post-operative discomfort, and helps to maintain the relationship of the soft tissue flap to the underlying bone. In situations where it is felt desirable to apically reposition the flap in order to maximise pocket reduction, then it is necessary to reflect the flap beyond the mucogingival junction so that it is free to adopt a new relationship without any tension.

Following apical repositioning a continuous suture is used, independently suspending the buccal and lingual flaps around the teeth. They can therefore adopt independent and different relationships to the teeth and bone margin. In order to prevent an apically displaced flap from moving coronally, a periodontal pack is placed. In many cases, however, interrupted sutures can be used and a pack is optional (see fig. 9).

*Postoperative care and instructions*

1. Toothbrushing and interdental cleaning of the surgical area should be avoided.

2. Chlorhexidine mouthwash should be used twice or more daily for one minute.

3. Post-operative swelling is normally minimal. A cold compress or ice bag should be applied to the outside of the face.

4. Analgesics should be taken as required. It is normal to have post-operative discomfort during the first 36 to 48 hours.

5. Post-operative bleeding should be controlled by local pressure. A swab moistened with chlorhexidine mouthwash is ideal.

6. Smokers are advised to stop for at least one week.

7. A soft diet is essential. Acidic or spicy foods are best avoided.

8. Systemic antibiotics are not usually indicated unless there has been a lot of bone recontouring or the patient has had problems with post-operative infections in the past.

## Summary and conclusions

Results from comparative surgical studies have shown small differences between methods when evaluated over a few years post-surgically. Early interim results suggest that apical repositioning is more effective at reducing probing depth, replaced flaps (such as the modified Widman technique) offer slight advantages in terms of gain in clinical attachment, and procedures which involve extensive bone removal or exposure result in more bone loss and loss of attachment. The replaced flaps should in theory produce better aesthetics than the apical repositioned flap. In the long term however, the former tend to recede slightly whilst there is some coronal rebound in the latter, thereby producing relatively little difference between them when good plaque control is maintained.

In all procedures there is loss in height of the interdental tissues, even if the labial tissue is maintained, and this can be aesthetically displeasing to some individuals. However it should also be remembered that effective non-surgical treatment can result in similar changes in tissue height and contour, and there is no guarantee of preservation of pre-existing dentogingival aesthetics. All routine periodontal treatment results in gingival shrinkage to some degree.

In many cases periodontal surgery will, in reality, involve a combination of replacement, apical repositioning and resection due to the uneven pattern of disease and different anatomical constraints of the palate, tuberosities and retromolar regions. This is shown in figure 12.

In summary the surgical procedures should:
1. Produce well contoured flaps of even thickness which are tailored to the shape of the

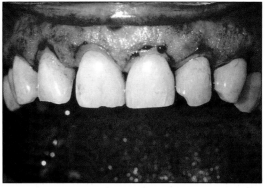
(a)

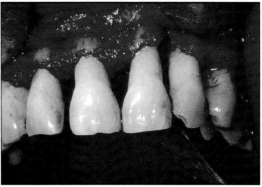
(b)

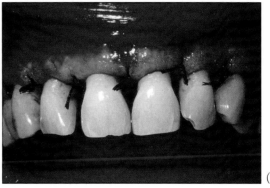
(c)

**Fig. 12** (a) Relatively normal gingival contour in upper incisor region despite quite extensive pocketing. (b) The same area following elevation of flaps and removal of soft tissue showing uneven bone contour and presence of infrabony lesion at upper right lateral incisor region. Note the variation in distance between the cement enamel junction and crestal bone at different sites. (c) Flap secured with interrupted sutures. Note that the gingival margin is apical to that which existed preoperatively. This is mainly due to some excision of tissue in the inverse bevel incision and collapsing in of the flap margins interdentally. At some sites the flap will just cover the bone crest by about 2 mm and a normal dentogingival junction would be established quite rapidly. In the region of the deep infrabony lesion considerable healing and maturation will have to take place to repair this void.

tooth surfaces and permit good coverage of the alveolar bone and any bone defects.

2. Provide good access to the root surfaces by direct and indirect vision to allow root planing of disease affected surfaces which remain subgingival at the end of the procedure.

3. Allow some recontouring of bone if this is necessary to allow good flap adaptation.

Surgical procedures should:
1 Produce well contoured flaps of even thickness which are tailored to the shape of the tooth surfaces and permit good coverage of the alveolar bone and any bone defects.
2 Provide good access to the root surfaces by direct and indirect vision to allow root planing of disease affected surfaces which remain subgingival at the end of the procedure.
3 Allow some recontouring of bone if this is necessary to allow good flap adaptation.
4 Produce good stabilisation of flap margins by careful suturing and packing if required.
5 Allow rapid post-operative healing and re-establishment of the patients' plaque control as soon as possible.

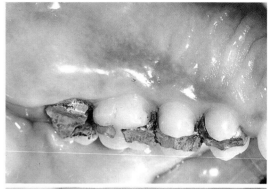

(a)

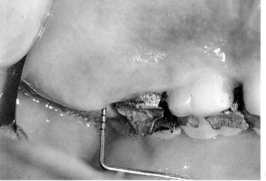

(b

**Fig. 13**

4. Produce good stabilisation of flap margins by careful suturing and packing if required.

5. Allow rapid post-operative healing and re-establishment of the patient's plaque control as soon as possible.

There are many differences between treatment of anterior and posterior teeth. Results from numerous trials have uniformly described less favourable results with posterior teeth using both surgical and non-surgical treatment. This is due to molar teeth being:
1. Involved with more complex disease.
2. Having more difficult root morphology.
3. Having poorer access for both clinician and patient.

Treatment of molar teeth therefore is much more difficult and will be considered in more detail in the next chapter.

## Surgical management of the palate and tuberosity

Periodontal surgery in the palate and distal to the last standing molar deserves special consideration and is an area which many clinicians find difficult to manage. The most important factors to appreciate are:
1. The tissue is thicker than other areas and usually more firmly bound down to the underlying bone.
2. Access can be difficult.
3. Pocket reduction/elimination has to be achieved with resective techniques. It is not possible to compensate for inaccurate flap design by apical or coronal repositioning.

In order to compensate for these difficulties the following basic recommendations are given:
1. Make sure the incision is firmly down to bone and through periosteum. Start the elevation at a point where it is easy to verify that you have exposed palatal bone and work from this point using the bone and not the teeth as a fulcrum point. If in doubt repeat the incision.
2. Adjust the head rest to tilt the patient's head backwards and ask the patient to rotate their head to allow direct vision of the area by the operator.

3. Judgement of the shape and position of the outline incision is difficult, but can be made easier by reflecting the full thickness of the palate through a crevicular incision. The morphology of the bone margin and roots can be seen and the outline incision made accordingly. This technique is illustrated in the following case.

*Preoperative description*
Figure 13 shows the palatal view of the maxillary molar and premolar teeth. The gingival margin has not receded and there is considerable enlargement on the palatal aspect of the second molar and the tuberosity. In this area there is a large degree of false pocketing. Examination with a probe demonstrates a probing depth of at least 7 mm on the distal aspect (fig. 13b). The amalgam restoration in the second molar extends subgingivally and is in need of replacement.

*The incisions and flap reflection*
The incision is started at the tuberosity (fig. 14). A number 12 blade has been used to incise from the distal point of the tuberosity anteriorly to the mid-point of the distal surface of the second molar. The incision is extended from the distal crevice around to the palatal crevices firmly down to bone. Incision into the distal crevice is best accomplished with a specialised periodontal knife, such as a buck knife. A subsequent incision is made at right angles to this (running

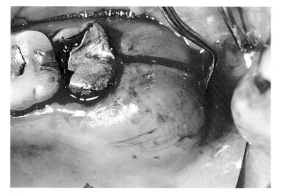

**Fig. 14**

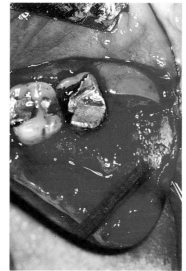
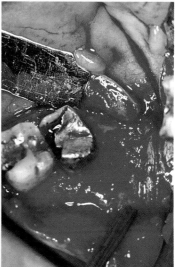

**Fig. 15**                              **Fig. 16**

bucco-palatally) at the distal aspect of the tuberosity with a Goldman Fox gingivectomy knife.

The palatal flap is reflected from the teeth and extending to the palatal part of the tuberosity (fig. 15). The flaps should reflect relatively easily provided the incision has not inadvertently extended into an infrabony defect. The exposed bone has a number of small exostoses (arrow). The buccal incision utilises a standard inverse bevel incision from the distobuccal line angle of the second molar continuing anteriorly.

The buccal flap and buccal tuberosity are reflected (fig. 16). The pocket lining is removed from the buccal aspect together with soft tissue tags between the teeth and palatally. All inflammatory tissue is curetted from within bone defects. This ensures good access to the root surfaces for planing with hand and ultrasonic instruments.

The next stage is to trim and thin the palatal and tuberosity flaps to eliminate the pocketing and provide good bone coverage and adaptation to the tooth surfaces.

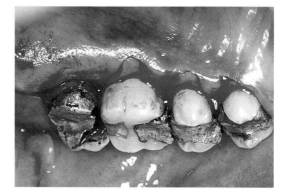

**Fig. 17**

*The palatal flap*

Having inspected the shape of the root surfaces and the level of the alveolar bone, the palatal flap is replaced and an outline incision (depth 1 to 2 mm) made to conform with the underlying morphology. Figure 17 shows an exaggerated scalloped incision which is designed to maximise interdental coverage by shaping 'papillae'.

The next stage is to thin the palatal flap (fig. 18). A new 15 blade is introduced into the outline incision and worked apically with a filleting action. The palatal tissue is relatively stable compared with a buccal flap but does require some support for this thinning incision to be made. It is therefore recommended that the operator supports the flap with a finger (fig. 19). In this way the palatal flap is supported between the flat surface of the scalpel blade and the finger. The incision is continued to a point where the excised tissue is freed from the flap.

The planes of the outline (O) and thinning (T) incisions are shown in the diagram of a

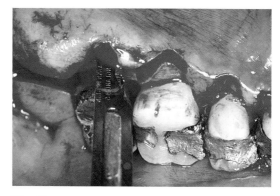

**Fig. 18**

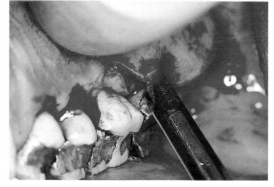

**Fig. 19**

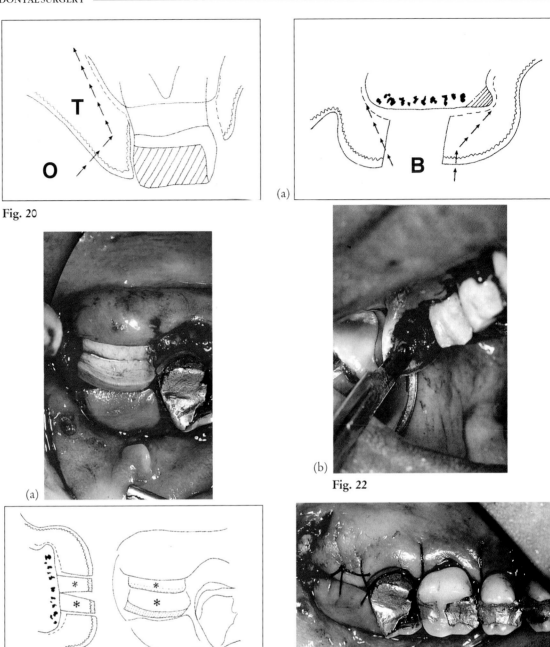

Fig. 20

(a)

(a)

(b)

Fig. 22

(b)

Fig. 21

Fig. 23

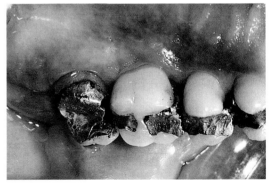

Fig. 24

bucco-palatal section through the second molar (fig. 20).

## The tuberosity

The thick fibrous tuberosity flaps are thinned and shortened (fig. 21). The wedges of excess tissue incised from both the palatal and buccal flaps are shown and marked with an asterisk. Figure 22a represents a bucco-palatal section through the tuberosity region. The line on the buccal side (B) depicts thinning of the buccal flap. The line on the palatal side depicts shortening and thinning of the palatal flap. The shaded area (*) represents the bony exostoses which may be smoothed off to allow better flap adaptation. The thinning of the buccal tuberosity flap

is facilitated if it can be supported between a mirror head (fig. 22b) or the operators finger (as with the palate in fig. 19) and the scalpel blade.

*Suturing*

The trimmed flaps are sutured (fig. 23). The tuberosity flaps are closed with one interrupted suture distally and as part of a continuous suture which closes the flaps around the teeth.

*Healing*

Figure 24 shows the area after 20 days of healing. The level of the palatal gingival margin is more apical and the margin of the amalgam in the second molar is clearly visible.

# Instruments for periodontal surgery

This series of photographs (figs 25–31) shows a typical set of surgical instruments and their uses. There are many other instruments available but the authors have found that these relatively basic sets are sufficient to undertake the majority of simple and advanced periodontal surgical techniques.

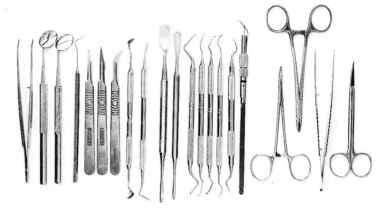

**Fig. 25** A set of periodontal surgical instruments comprising form left to right: College tweezers; 2 dental mirrors; Periodontal probe; 3 scalpel handles preloaded with blade numbers 15, 11 and 12, it improves efficiency to have at least two types of blade pre-loaded; 2 Gingivectomy knives — Goldman Fox numbers 7 and 11 (see fig. 26); 2 Periosteal elevators/retractors — Prichard PR3 and Dial number 9; Large surgical curette — Prichard PR1 (see fig. 27); 3 smaller surgical curettes — Goldman Fox numbers 2, 3 and 4 (see fig. 27); Rhodes chisel (see fig. 28); Ultrasonic tip — Cavitron P10; Fine curved mosquito forceps; Needle holders — box joint (tungsten carbide tipped); Tissue forceps — Fine rat toothed; Surgical scissors — Fine curved with one serrated blade (tungsten carbide tipped).

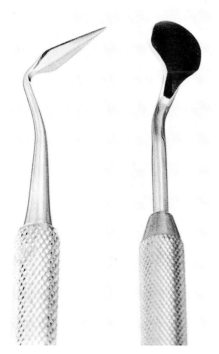

**Fig. 26** Golman Fox periodontal knives no. 7 ('kidney shaped') and no. 11 (pointed blade). Both instruments have angled blades, facilitating access to more difficult areas. These instruments are kept sharp with sharpening stones and should be used as a scalpel (not a curette). Number 7 is particularly suitable for tuberosity incisions (See section Palate and tuberosity). The no. 11 is generally used for crevicular incisions in inaccessible areas. These instruments were originally designed for the gingivectomy procedure, no. 7 for the bulk of the excision and no. 11 interproximally.

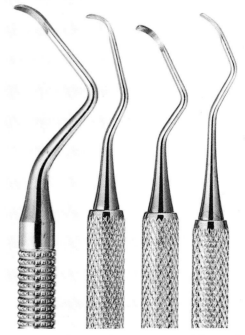

**Fig. 27** A set of surgical curettes. From left to right: Prichard PR1 — Large broad tipped general purpose surgical curette; Golman Fox 2 — Long terminal shank with angled blade tip similar in configuration to the Gracey 1/2 but more robust; Goldman Fox 3 — Universal curette shape with long terminal shank and curved tip; Golman Fox 4 — Universal curette shape with shorter terminal shank and flatter tip.

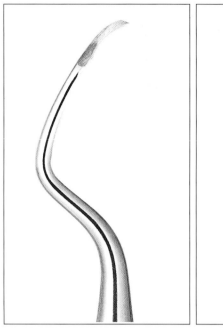
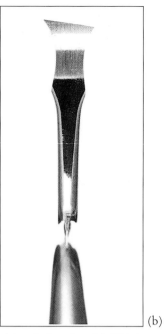

(a)                                                                    (b)

**Fig. 28** Rhodes chisel viewed from side (a) and plan view (b). This is a 'pull-action' chisel used both for bone (see also fig. 29) and soft tissue removal, particularly in the tuberosity flap procedure when the broad curved blade facilitates removal of the soft tissue wedges distal to the last molar.

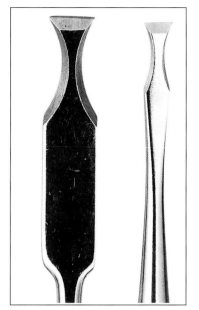

**Fig. 30** Enlarged views of the working tips of the Ochsenbien (left) and TG0 (right) chisels.

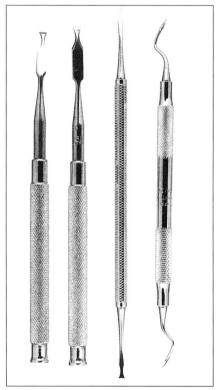

**Fig. 29** Surgical bone chisels. From left to right: Pair of Ochsenbien chisels (OCH1 and OCH2) — in this view the cutting edges are curved away from and towards observer; Mini Ochsenbien chisel (TG0) — a smaller double ended version of the above; Rhodes chisel 36/37 (see fig. 28).

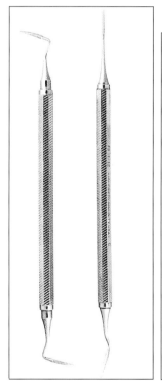
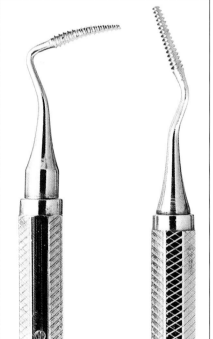

**Fig 31** Interproximal bone files. These are double 'safe-sided' instruments for the reduction of bone height interproximally: Schluger file — curved blades; Buck file FB 11/12 — straight blades.

# 5

# Treatment of multi-rooted teeth

This chapter covers:
1 Furcation grading
2 Treatment options

It should be clear from the previous chapters that posterior teeth present particular difficulties in both non-surgical and surgical management. Furcation involvement is obviously encountered more frequently in moderate to advanced periodontitis. However, some patients with relatively early attachment loss may have furcation involvement. This is particularly the case with short root trunks (ie the distance between the cement–enamel junction and the furcation entrance) and the presence of enamel spurs (or more rarely enamel pearls) extending into the furcation area. In addition, upper first premolars usually have a concavity on the mesial aspect of the crown (the canine fossa) which extends apically to the furcation area and if gingival recession occurs may present problems with plaque control.

In most patients the deepest pocketing is seen on the proximal surfaces of the teeth and it is on these surfaces that the mesial and distal furcation entrances of upper molars and first premolars are located. They are generally more difficult to detect than buccal/lingual furcation entrances. Careful clinical and radiographic evaluation is essential in determining the degree of involvement and treatment possibilities. In general when evaluating the molar series of teeth it should be remembered that from first to second to third molar:
1 The roots gets progressively shorter
2 The space between the roots is smaller and fusion of roots is more common
3 The roots divide more apically — longer root trunk
4 Endodontics and restorative management become more difficult
5 Access by both patient and operator is more difficult.

For a given level of disease, the more distal the molar is in the series, the worse the prognosis and the more difficult the treatment. In addition, the two-rooted upper first premolar usually presents special difficulties with management because of its unfavourable root morphology and because its loss has important aesthetic implications.

## Assessment

Furcation involvement should be evaluated at the diagnostic appointment, during non-surgical treatment, and at surgery. Identification of the full extent of disease affecting molar teeth is very difficult when one considers the complexity and inaccessibility of the internal aspects of the furcation area. To take this to its logical extreme, the most accurate assessment of individual roots of a multirooted tooth would only be possible by vertical probing around their circumference following removal of the crown to the level at which the roots are separate. This type of evaluation has been recommended when preservation of a single root from a molar is critical to a proposed restorative treatment plan. For the most part however we rely on horizontal grading of the furcation (fig. 1), vertical probing depths and radiographic examination. It is quite obvious that each of these assessments will occasionally detect an involvement that another will miss (fig. 2).

Due to the anatomy of upper molars the mesial furcation entrance is located nearer the palate and the distal furcation nearer the buccal aspect. It is therefore usually easier to examine these furcation entrances from the respective aspects.

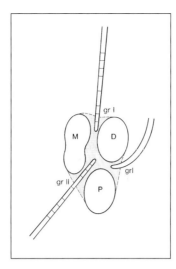

**Fig. 1** Furcation grading: diagrammatic representation of an upper molar furcation with straight and curved probes demonstrating:
Grade I    just detectable (less than 3 mm horizontally)
Grade II   Substantial involvement (over 3 mm and within the central part of the furcation)
Grade III Through and through involvement
(M = mesial, D = distal, P = palatal roots)

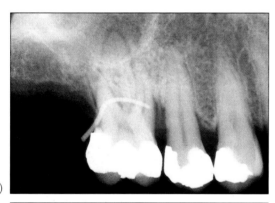

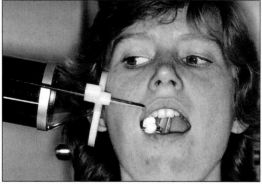

**Fig. 2** (a) Radiograph of an upper molar with a gutta percha point placed in the furcation from mesial to distal demonstrating the now obvious grade III involvement which was difficult to examine clinically and not previously observable radiographically. Good quality long cone parallel radiographs with minimum distortion and without superimposition of anatomical structures such as the zygomatic arch are essential. (b) Patient with Rinn holder in place, supported by cottonwool rolls, and long cone tube directed along the aiming arm.

Specially designed fine furcation probes are the best instruments for clinical detection of furcation entrances, but examination with a universal curette will also give a good idea as to whether the furcation is instrumentable. It may be surprising to learn that a large proportion of molar furcation entrances are smaller than the width of a fine curette and are thus impossible to clean without enlarging the furcation entrance. On occasions an endodontic lesion on a molar may masquerade as a periodontal furcation involvement. If in an otherwise periodontally healthy mouth a single molar has a furcation involvement, then an endodontic lesion should first be considered as the cause, followed by anatomical variations such as enamel projections or pearls.

## Treatment options

The basic treatment options will now be considered in turn.

Treatment options
1   Extraction
2   Root planing
3   Surgery
    3.1 Open root planing
    3.2 Reshaping the furcation entrance: the furcation operation
    3.3 Making a tunnel
4   Advanced surgery involving removal of roots
    4.1 Root resection
    4.2 Hemisection
5   Guided tissue regeneration and grafting (see article 6: Regenerative and reconstructive periodontal treatment)

*Extraction*

This treatment option is more easily applied to second and third molars and especially to those that are overerupted or unopposed. Aesthetics and function are generally satisfied with a shortened dental arch extending from first molar to first molar. In some individuals it is acceptable to lose first molars and even premolars without provision of replacements. In the case that other treatment options are viable, for example hemisection or root resection, due consideration should be given to the prognosis of the adjacent teeth before condemning a tooth to extraction. Extraction is more likely to be considered when the tooth has:
1   A poor restorative/endodontic status
2   Root caries
3   Given symptoms such as repeated periodontal abscesses

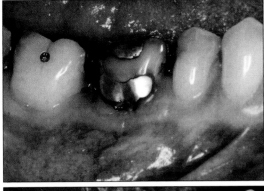

(a)

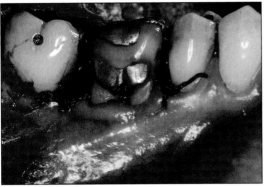

(b)

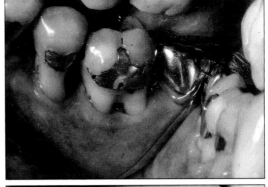

(a)

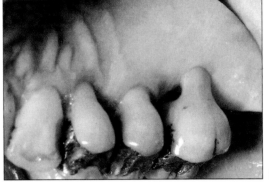

(b)

**Fig. 3** Lower molar buccal furcation (a) before and (b) after reshaping with high speed finishing burs. The horizontal depth of the furcation has been reduced by tooth surface reduction and reshaping the buccal alveolar bone crest to allow formation of a papilla within the furcation entrance.

**Fig. 4** (a) A tunnel preparation in a lower molar which had a grade III furcation involvement. The concavities within this long tunnel are reduced by reshaping the furcation with burs, but in many cases residual concave surfaces make the tooth susceptible to root caries. (b) A tunnel preparation between the remaining two roots of an upper molar, the third root having been resected. In this situation the tunnel is shorter and there are fewer concavities allowing more effective plaque control by the patient.

4   Proved impossible for the patient to keep free of plaque

5   Shown progressive loss of clinical attachment and bone and/or increasing mobility

6   No strategic value in terms of aesthetics, function or as a potential abutment.

Explanation of these factors is more likely to result in agreement of this treatment option by the patient. It is a salutatory experience to examine an extracted molar following failure of treatment to see how complex the furcation anatomy is and the ease with which a nidus of plaque and calculus can remain undisturbed.

*Root planing*

This method of treatment was dealt with in article 2 and constraints of treatment of molar teeth explained. Whereas grade I furcations are often readily instrumentable, the inner aspects of grade II and grade III are usually technically impossible to render free of plaque. Remember that in most cases root planing will involve some degree of reshaping of the furcation entrance.

*Surgery*

Surgery has a great advantage in providing better access to and visibility of the furcation. In advanced involvement however, there are likely to be surfaces which are still impossible to

reach. Access to furcations can be improved by reshaping the entrance (fig. 3) and instrumentation of difficult surfaces may also be accomplished with rotary instruments which is only possible when a flap has been raised. In grade III furcations on two rooted molars the furcation can sometimes be reshaped to allow better access by the patient. This is referred to as a tunnel preparation and is illustrated in figure 4. Tunnel preparations need widely spaced roots, short root trunks and meticulous cleaning/fluoride applications to reduce the chance of failure due to root caries or recurrent periodontitis.

*Advanced surgery involving removal of roots*

This type of surgery is performed relatively infrequently. It is technically demanding and expensive. It is most readily applied to first molars where one root has lost a great deal of support compared with the remaining roots. Removing a root obviously involves endodontic considerations and the resulting weakening of the crown requires restorative considerations. This type of surgery is best explained by illustrations from two cases in figures 5 and 6.

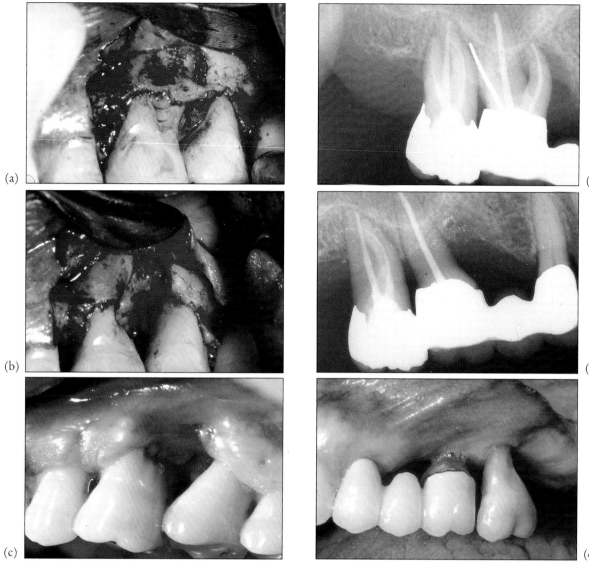

**Fig. 5** (a) Clinical photograph of an upper first molar following elevation of a flap, showing severe bone loss around the distobuccal root. A grade III furcation involvement was detected clinically from the buccal to the distal furcation. (b) Resection of the distobuccal root has been carried out with a high speed bur and the undersurface of the crown re-shaped to produce a smooth 'flowing' contour. It is very important to avoid leaving small spurs and ridges by incomplete resection and shaping. The buccal wall of the socket has been reduced to facilitate extraction of the root and to allow 'collapsing in' of the flap, thereby providing a gingival contour and dentogingival junction which is easy for the patient to keep free of plaque. (c) One week post-operative.

The decision to resect a root from a molar tooth is always a difficult one, and should only be contemplated if the prognosis of the tooth will be predictably improved. In order to be more assured of this, it is often better to perform routine access surgery so that a direct evaluation of the furcation involvement is possible. The clinician needs to visualise what the morphology of the defect will be following the removal of a root and, particularly, the level of attach-

**Fig. 6** (a) Clinical and (b) radiographic illustrations of root resections on teeth used to support bridges. Both first and second molars had been root treated. Surgery involved removal of both buccal roots of the first molar, the mesial of which had lost its entire support. The distobuccal root was resected from the second molar. (c) The clinical apperance from the buccal aspect post-treatment.

ment, bone and residual furcation problem at the remaining roots. This has to be considered together with any restorative or endodontic difficulties.

Having made the decision that a root resection would be the treatment of choice, there are two options as to when this procedure can be performed:

1. At the time of the initial access surgery providing the patient has been fully informed. The vital pulp exposure can be capped with calcium hydroxide and a restorative material in an attempt to preserve pulp vitality. Alternatively the pulp can be left exposed and root canal treatment started within 2 weeks. The decision to carry out a root resection is always easier if the tooth has an existing successful root filling.

2. The root resection can be postponed until root canal treatment has been performed on the roots which are to remain. Under these circumstances it is helpful to fill the coronal part of the root to be resected with a material such as amalgam so that a restoration is in place at the time of resection.

Successful treatment relies upon an accurate diagnosis and competent treatment in a number of disciplines, and failure can result from a number of causes.

Causes of failure of advanced treatment modalities
1   Recurrent periodontitis resulting from:
    Misdiagnosis
    Failure to adequately instrument or reshape area
    Poor oral hygiene
2   Endodontic or combined endodontic/periodontitis
3   Caries (usually root caries)
4   Tooth fracture

## Conclusions

The range of treatment alternatives for molar teeth is wide, but application of the more sophisticated procedures is relatively limited. Molar teeth with advanced furcation involvement can often be kept in function for many years, given good levels of maintenance care by both clinician and patient. They are however, the most common teeth to be lost due to periodontal disease and are too often involved in complex restorative treatment plans without adequate treatment or evaluation.

# 6 Reconstructive periodontal treatment

This chapter covers:
1 Periodontal ligament regeneration
2 Gingival recession and attached gingiva

Regeneration of the lost tissues of the periodontium is an ideal goal and the subject of much research and ingenious clinical techniques. Reconstructive or regenerative techniques are used either singly or in combination for two main purposes: (1) to regain lost periodontal ligament attachment and (2) to provide a wider zone of attached gingiva.

## Periodontal ligament regeneration

Regeneration involves reformation of cementum, bone and an intervening fibrous tissue, the periodontal ligament, attached to the mineralised tissues by Sharpey's fibres. A simple way to appreciate the events involved would be to consider the healing of an infrabony pocket treated by replaced flap surgery (see chapter 4) and to consider how this may be modified (fig. 1).

Preservation of soft tissue flaps which are closely approximated to the tooth surfaces should give maximum protection to the underlying clot and connective tissues. The clot acts as a glue between the flap, tooth surface and underlying tissues and acts as a scaffold for the healing process. Organisation of the clot by proliferating capillaries and fibroblasts occurs rapidly from adjacent gingival connective tissue, bone and periodontal ligament.

Initially the alveolar bone undergoes resorption, which is more pronounced following prolonged exposure, surgical recontouring and inflammatory changes. The gingival epithelium rapidly divides and migrates on the connective tissue aspect of the flap to eventually contact the tooth surface and form a junctional epithelium. This rapid migration has been held responsible for the prevention of a connective tissue attachment.

Cell division, migration, differentiation, adhesion, matrix deposition, organisation and compartmentalisation in this process are extremely complex. These factors are only simplistically addressed in current therapeutic procedures. Traditionally the types of defects which show the best response to conventional treatment are deep and narrow with large areas of surrounding bone and periodontal ligament. These defects have been classified variously as intrabony, infrabony or '3-wall' and also show the best response to regenerative techniques. Conversely, broad defects with only one remaining bone wall have unfavourable regenerative potential. The most challenging area is supracrestal regeneration where the destructive process has resulted in horizontal bone and attachment loss.

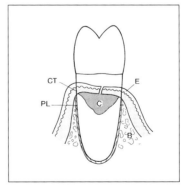

**Fig. 1** Diagram of infrabony defect treated by flap surgery showing good coverage by the flap and potential tissue contributions to the area from epithelium (E), gingival connective tissue (CT), alveolar bone (B) and periodontal ligament (PL). The defect is initially filled with blood clot (C). Optimum results can only be achieved if the affected root surface has been meticulously instrumented, and subsequently kept free of plaque.

Because of variable and unpredictable clinical results many attempts have been made to improve this process. These are listed here and will be considered in turn.

Procedures used to enhance regeneration
1 Bone and bone-substitute grafting to fill the defect
2 Prevention/retardation of epithelial downgrowth
  (a) Root surface conditioning
  (b) Guided tissue regeneration using non-resorbable and resorbable membranes to also exclude other unwanted cells
3 Growth factor application to promote specific cell proliferation and differentiation

### Bone grafting

Bone loss and repair are normally assessed radiographically, although some research studies have employed surgical re-entry procedures. There is no doubt that bone repair can occur following those non-surgical and simple surgical treatments which effectively eliminate inflammation (fig. 2). Grafting with bone and bone substitutes to enhance this repair process has been a popular procedure and is currently experiencing a revival/reappraisal.

An increased radiodensity will result from the placement of a graft material (particularly if mineralised) into a bone defect. This will produce a radiographic improvement if the measuring system is sufficiently sophisticated. Synthetic materials which are non-resorbable, such as dense particulate hydroxyapatite, are incorporated in the healing tissue and are eventually surrounded by mature fibrous tissue and variable amounts of bone formation. The material should be viewed as a space filler with little inductive properties.

Bioactive glasses have been shown to bond to bone and soft tissues and provide very good space maintenance. Other forms of calcium phosphate/hydroxyapatite are resorbable and may be more bone inductive. Bone repair following grafting with both resorbable and non-resorbable synthetic materials is unfortunately no more predictable than an ungrafted defect, although the former often show radiographic advantages.

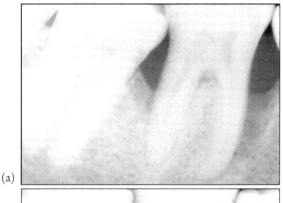

(a)

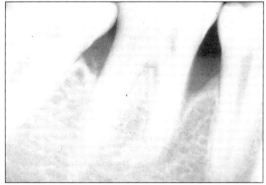

(b)

Fig. 2 (a) Radiograph of bone defect prior to treatment. (b) Bone fill after treatment.

Grafts of autogenous bone are best. Bone can be obtained from intraoral sites using small trephines, burs or chisels, with little additional discomfort to the patient. The amount of bone available is usually limited and the need to obtain larger quantities led some clinicians to use the hip as a donor site. This is a painful procedure for the patient and early experience using fresh hip grafts showed a high potential for resorption and ankylosis of the teeth. Freezing the hip marrow graft largely overcame this latter problem.

However, the desire to avoid major surgery for the procurement of sufficient bone graft material has led to the utilisation of bone bank material. This graft material, which is particularly popular in the USA for use in periodontal surgery and augmentation for implants, is obtained from human donors screened for blood-borne diseases, and thoroughly treated to render it safe and non-antigenic. The material is freeze dried and either mineralised or demineralised. Bone proteins within the material are effective at inducing new bone formation.

Repair of bone within a periodontal defect is a good sign, regardless of the procedure used, as it indicates a marked reduction of inflammation. It has been demonstrated in animal models and limited human histological material, however, that despite the appearance of a relatively normal radiographic periodontal ligament space, the attachment to the root surface is a long junctional epithelium with a narrow zone of connective tissue between it and newly formed bone. This is taken as evidence that epithelialisation of the root surface is a major factor preventing formation of a connective tissue attachment. It could also be viewed as a protection against formation of a bony ankylosis/resorption.

### Prevention/retardation of epithelial downgrowth

ROOT SURFACE DEMINERALISATION
Demineralisation of planed root surfaces exposes collagen fibrils and may enhance initial adhesion of the connective tissue of the flap and subsequently allow formation of a collagen fibre linkage. Early animal experiments using citric acid (pH 1) also demonstrated an accelerated cementogenesis and therefore true connective tissue attachment. Subsequent trials failed to substantiate this and healing was more likely to result in root resorption. Currently, there is still considerable interest in this area utilising tetracycline solutions which are both demineralising and antibacterial with useful substantivity.

GUIDED TISSUE REGENERATION
In a now classic series of experimental animal models it was shown that the residual periodontal ligament is the most likely tissue to contain

cells capable of regenerating a new periodontal ligament attachment. During healing of a periodontal defect, guided tissue regeneration aims to provide conditions which facilitate ingrowth of cells from the ligament whilst excluding those derived from epithelium and gingival connective tissue. The surgical procedure is therefore modified to allow placement of an exclusionary membrane between the meticulously instrumented root surface and the overlying flap (fig. 3). The procedure is illustrated in figure 4.

Ideally the membrane should form a small tent over the defect to provide sufficient space to accommodate the missing tissues. Organisation of the clot is therefore limited to contributions from the periodontal ligament and alveolar bone. Whereas it was initially postulated that the appropriate progenitor cells were present solely in the periodontal ligament, it now seems that cells within the bone may also contribute to the formation of the ligament/cementum. Although ankylosis is theoretically possible, in practice it does not seem to occur and the improvements in attachment levels have been attributed to regeneration, although little histological proof is available in human specimens.

Most clinical success to date has been recorded with non-resorbable membranes made of e-PTFE (Gore-Tex). This material has to be removed 4 to 6 weeks after the initial surgical procedure, requiring a second operation and healing period. This has led to the development of resorbable membranes, which are made of synthetic materials such as polyglactin (the same material as some sutures eg vicryl) or from animal or human proteins such as collagen or demineralised sheets of cortical bone. The physical properties of some of these materials make them difficult to handle clinically and there are few if any published trials reporting their efficacy in periodontal or bone regenerative treatment.

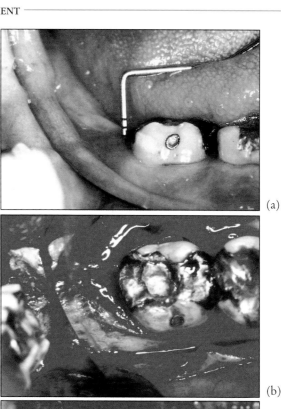

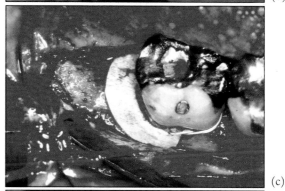

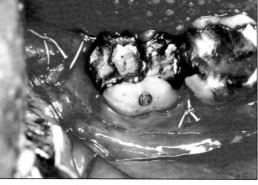

Fig. 4 (a) A probe examining a deep pocket distal to a lower molar. (b) The site after surgical exposure showing a large bone defect. (c) Following extensive root planing and removal of inflammatory tissue the defect is covered with a Gore-Tex membrane which is secured with a suture. (d) The membrane is completely covered with the flap and left buried for 4 to 6 weeks.

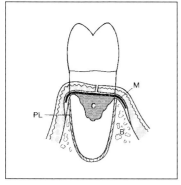

Fig. 3 Diagram of infrabony defect as shown in figure 1 showing placement of an exclusionary membrane (M) to prevent contributions by epithelium and gingival connective tissue whilst allowing periodontal ligament (PL) and bone (B) to grow into the area.

Most published trials with e-PTFE membranes report a small advantage over control surgical sites. Many of the best results are collections of case reports without controls. The procedure does produce some very good clinical results but more research is required to define which defects and patients would benefit most from this treatment and how well results are maintained in the long term. Given that resorbable membranes prove to be equally effective then they will certainly be more cost effective and may enjoy wider use.

GROWTH FACTORS

This is a rapidly developing field which has had few clinical trials. Freeze-dried bone is probably effective because of high levels of osteogenic proteins such as the bone morphogenetic proteins. Periodontal ligament fibroblast proliferation may be enhanced by growth factors such as PDGF (platelet derived growth factor) and insulin-like growth factor. Early experiments in animal models have shown promise. Techniques are available to mass produce growth factors, and technology is being developed to allow slow release over sufficient time periods to promote success.

*Conclusion*

The quest for more predictable regeneration has led some clinicians to combine treatment procedures such as acid demineralisation of the root surface, grafting with freeze dried bone and covering the defect with an exclusionary membrane. Very promising results have been published with these techniques but it is far from clear what the optimum combinations are in any given situation.

# Gingival recession and attached gingiva

Gingival recession occurs with chronic periodontitis as a result of the disease process and as a consequence of successful treatment. However, this section will consider localised gingival recession usually resulting from direct trauma to thin gingival tissue or more rarely from plaque-induced inflammatory damage. It is a common concern for patients who often believe that it may lead to tooth loss, which fortunately is an unlikely event.

Gingival recession may produce an aesthetic problem (particularly in the upper anterior teeth) or it may result in a diminution in the width of keratinised/attached gingiva. There is considerable debate as to what constitutes an adequate width of attached gingiva from a functional/biological view.

It is obviously important to address the patient's complaint and to determine the importance of the physical features in relationship to it.

Patients' concerns
1 Tooth loss
2 Appearance
3 Sensitivity to hot and cold
4 Gingival soreness or bleeding
5 Will it progress?

Examination of gingival recession and associated mucogingival problems
1 Tooth involved and aesthetic implications
2 Measurement of recession
— CEJ to gingival margin
— width of recession
3 Probing depth and presence of pocketing
4 Width of keratinised gingiva — gingival margin to mucogingival junction
— subtract probing depth to give width of attached gingiva
5 Functional inadequacy of attached gingiva is present if:
— gingival margin pulls away from tooth surface when tension applied to mucosa (frenae may also be involved)
— the gingival/mucosal junction is continuously traumatised by patients oral hygiene efforts
— co-existing pockets extend beyond mucogingival junction
— there is measurable progression of recession
6 Pattern of bone loss
— interproximal height
— lateral extension of dehiscence further apically
7 Do not forget to examine the restorative/endodontic status of affected tooth:
— presence of abrasion cavities (+/- erosion)

*Treatment*

It is easiest to illustrate this by considering two surgical procedures, one designed to increase the width of the attached gingiva and the other to repair an area of gingival recession.

Indications for treatment of recession/lack of attached gingiva
1 Aesthetics
2 Recession and pocketing — simultaneous correction of pocket depth
3 Progressive recession
4 Improve anatomy
— to reduce progression
— to facilitate OH
— to correct appearance

FREE GINGIVAL GRAFT

This procedure is usually employed to produce a wider zone of attached/keratinised gingiva without necessarily altering the position of the gingival margin. It is illustrated in figure 5. It involves transplantation of a graft of connective tissue covered by epithelium from the palate to a recipient site. The graft initially survives by diffusion of plasma from the recipient bed and

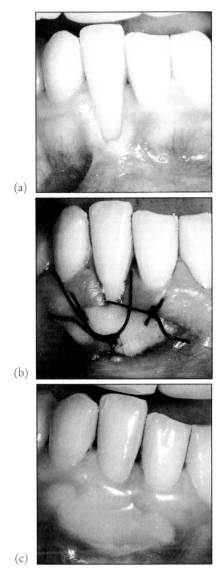

(a)

(b)

(c)

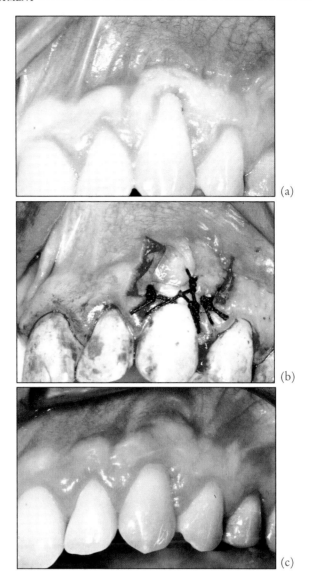

(a)

(b)

(c)

**Fig. 5** (a) A lower incisor with little keratinised gingiva and recession. (b) Following preparation of graft bed and suturing of free gingival graft taken from the palate. (c) Healed result after 1 year showing wide zone of attached keratinised gingiva and reduction of recession which has been helped by further 'creeping reattachment' of the gingival tissues.

**Fig. 6** (a) An upper canine with gingival recession presenting an aesthetic problem. (b) Papilla flaps have been rotated from the mesial and distal aspects to cover the defect. In addition, a connective tissue graft (taken from the palate) has been interposed between the flaps and the prepared root surface/ adjacent graft bed. (c) The healed result showing minimal recession and improvement in aesthetics.

the connective tissue dictates the type of epithelium growing on it.

PEDICLE GRAFT

Procedures which aim to repair areas of recession and thereby cover denuded root surfaces may be made more predictable by using a graft which maintains a blood supply ie a pedicle graft. This requires a suitable adjacent donor site which is itself going to be compromised by the procedure.

An example of this type of surgery is illustrated in figure 6. In this case it has been performed in combination with an inter-positional connective tissue graft taken from the palate to improve

the predictability. This is placed over the root surface and adjacent exposed bone and covered by the pedicles, which in this case are rotated from both sides of the tooth (double papilla flap).

## Conclusions

Regenerative techniques in periodontology are an exciting area of new developments based on good research and sound clinical practice. It is hoped that this chapter gives an idea of the range of techniques available and the type of situations where they are applicable.

# 7    Integrated treatment planning

**This chapter covers:**
1  **Treatment of drifted anterior teeth**
2  **Replacement of missing teeth**

The establishment of periodontal health should be a primary aim in all treatment plans. The methods by which this can be achieved have been dealt with in previous articles, but there are a number of situations where integration of these treatment methods with other dental disciplines needs to be clarified. To simplify matters this article will consider periodontal implications in two main areas: treatment of drifted anterior teeth and replacement of missing teeth.

## Treatment of drifted teeth

Drifting or spacing of the maxillary anterior teeth is a frequent complaint of patients with periodontitis and demands careful diagnostic evaluation before choosing the treatment options. This is because the cause of the problem is usually multifactorial. Therefore, the evaluation can be conveniently divided into three sections.

Evaluation of aetiology
1  Periodontal
2  Orthodontic
3  Restorative/occlusal

### Evaluation of aetiology

PERIODONTAL
In situations where occlusal or soft tissue forces are persistent and likely to produce movement of teeth, the required magnitude of force will be inversely proportional to the amount of periodontal support. Chronic periodontitis is the most common cause of destruction of the periodontal support. The pattern of attachment loss on an individual tooth is also pertinent. In many cases the deepest pocketing and the most severe bone loss is on the palatal aspect of a labially migrated incisor. This has led to the (unproven) proposal that the forces generated within the inflammatory lesion are responsible for the tooth movement. Recurrent abscesses in this situation however may lead to rapid destruction and drifting. The amount of periodontal support will also depend upon factors such as:

1. Root length.
2. Root shape eg very tapering root forms.
3. Root resorption eg post orthodontic.
4. Endodontic lesions destroying the apical periodontium.

These factors can only be accurately assessed by good quality intra-oral radiographs, which will also confirm the degree of bone loss estimated from the clinical probing examination. All these factors contribute to the mobility of the teeth which is further increased by inflammation and jiggling forces. Mobility, which can be seen or felt (by the clinician's fingers placed gently on the labial surface of the incisors) when the patient gently occludes, is known as fremitus and is an indication of jiggling.

ORTHODONTIC
It is important to establish whether the patient has previously had orthodontic correction of a class II division 1 incisor relationship which is no longer stable. Most individuals with drifting incisors (fig. 1) have a pre-existing tendency to this incisor relationship and incompetent lip morphology. In many cases it is only one or two of the incisors which escape the control of the lower lip and any tendency to lip bite will accentuate the situation. Other contributory parafunctional habits such as patients who persistently bite on a foreign object are more rarely encountered. At completion of the treatment

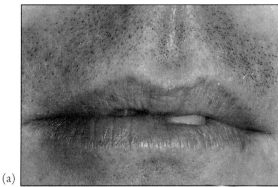

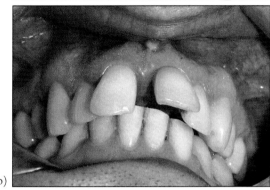

**Fig. 1** (a) and (b) Clinical photographs of drifted upper central incisors not within the control of the upper lip.

plan the incisors will need to be placed in a position of stability within the soft tissue pattern and adequate space is essential. This applies to space within the arch and careful consideration of the overbite which is often complete. It is prudent to seek the advice of an orthodontic specialist, particularly if repositioning is being considered.

### RESTORATIVE/OCCLUSAL

There are a number of potential restorative factors which may be associated with this problem.

1. Loss of posterior support causing the patient to function on the anterior teeth and often associated with forward posturing of the mandible.

2. Recent provision of anterior crowns which have altered the incisal guidance.

3. Occlusal interferences which may precipitate parafunctional activities.

The static and functional relationships of the teeth should be examined. It is particularly important to assess the incisal guidance and whether there is a marked horizontal discrepancy between the retruded contact position and the intercuspal position. The protrusive and lateral excursion contacts should be evaluated for fremitus and interferences (especially non-working).

### Treatment options

The treatment options should be more apparent after considering the above factors in addition to the obvious prognostic factors of the individual

teeth and dentition as a whole (see chapters 1 and 2). There are basically three options.

> Treatment options
> 1  Accept position of teeth
> 2  Orthodontic repositioning
> 3  Extraction and replacement

### ACCEPT POSITION OF TEETH

The position of the drifted teeth may be acceptable to the patient, particularly if the situation is unlikely to deteriorate further. Further drifting may be reduced with successful treatment of the periodontitis and occlusal factors. If the factors operating on the teeth are large then it is impos-

> Treatment of occlusal factors
> 1  Selective grinding to eliminate occlusal interferences and reduce fremitus
> 2  Replacement of unsatisfactory restorations
> 3  Provision of a posterior occlusion if possible and acceptable to patient
> 4  Provision of occlusal guard to dissipate parafunctional forces

sible to give the patient firm reassurance that the situation is stable. Many patients faced with the other options are prepared to accept the situation if the aesthetics are not too compromised.

### ORTHODONTIC REPOSITIONING

This is the most demanding of the treatment options and should not be entered into lightly. There are three basic guiding rules:

1. The periodontal condition must be treated initially.

2. The orthodontic forces have to be carefully controlled.

3. In most cases the orthodontic result will not be stable without permanent splinting.

Orthodontic tooth movement in untreated periodontitis is likely to result in further loss of attachment and in severe cases abscess formation and rapid destruction. The minimum periodontal treatment is thorough root planing and establishment of a high standard of supragingival plaque control by the patient. The provision of an orthodontic appliance may compromise plaque control and extra effort is required by the patient. If the orthodontic treatment is likely to be prolonged, then further subgingival instrumentation and maintenance treatment will be required during this phase.

In cases where periodontal surgery is required this can often be delayed until after the orthodontics has been completed. This has the advantage of re-establishing a dentogingival junction around the teeth in their corrected position, and subsequent maturation of the supracrestal collagen fibre arrangement may enhance stability.

While some simple cases can be managed with removable appliances, many will require fixed appliances and the services of a specialist orthodontist. In the latter case it is helpful if the orthodontist has had experience of moving teeth with compromised support. It is particularly important to avoid overloading and complications such as root resorption.

Most orthodontists will give no guarantee of stability of the end result in anything but the simplest of cases, and usually recommend permanent splinting. This is most predictably accomplished with full coverage restorations of the involved teeth but may need to be extended to involve a large number of teeth, eg from first premolar to first premolar. Splinting systems which rely on acid etch retained composite restorations may give adequate service in some instances. They range from simple wire and composite splints to Rochette and Maryland type retainers. These restorations are not as predictable as one would wish for such complex integrated treatment plans. Rochette frameworks have the advantage of being more easily removed if recementation is required.

Successful, predictable long-term retention is likely to need an extensive restoration. In some cases this is only achievable with conventional full coverage restorations. Under these circumstances due consideration needs to be given to extracting all or some of the drifted teeth in the first place. This may eliminate the need for orthodontics. Treatment of a patient involving orthodontics, periodontics and splinting is shown in figure 2.

## Replacement of missing teeth

Periodontal techniques can be usefully applied in the following areas:
1. Prior to provision of fixed bridge prostheses
    — crown lengthening
    — ridge augmentation.
2. Osseointegrated implant retained prostheses
    — guided bone regeneration
    — soft tissue augmentation.

### Prerestorative surgery

CROWN LENGTHENING
The periodontal surgical techniques described in article 4 can be usefully modified to:

1. Increase the clinical crown height to give adequate retention for crowns.

2. Expose subgingival restoration margins/secondary caries/fractures.

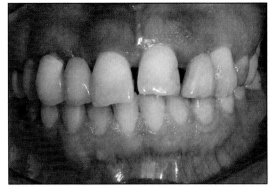

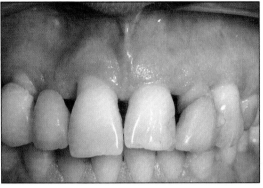

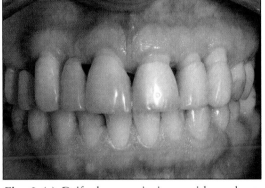

**Fig. 2** (a) Drifted upper incisors with moderate periodontitis. (b) Following non-surgical periodontal treatment and orthodontic repositioning. (c) Following periodontal surgery to eliminate residual pockets and splinting to maintain the result.

This procedure is illustrated in figure 3.

Severe attrition and erosion often lead to a situation where full coverage restoration of the teeth is necessary, but the available clinical crown height does not provide sufficient retention following preparation. In many individuals there is compensatory overeruption of the teeth. This also results in the dentogingival junction moving with the tooth, together with the alveolar bone, whereas the mucogingival junction maintains its level. The net result is an increase in the width of the keratinised/attached gingiva and maintenance of the pre-existing biological width (fig. 3b). Removal of soft tissues and underlying bone is necessary to achieve an increase in the height of the clinical crown. Where there has been periodontal pocketing the amount of soft tissue resection is determined by pocket depth, width of keratinised gingiva and the extra crown height

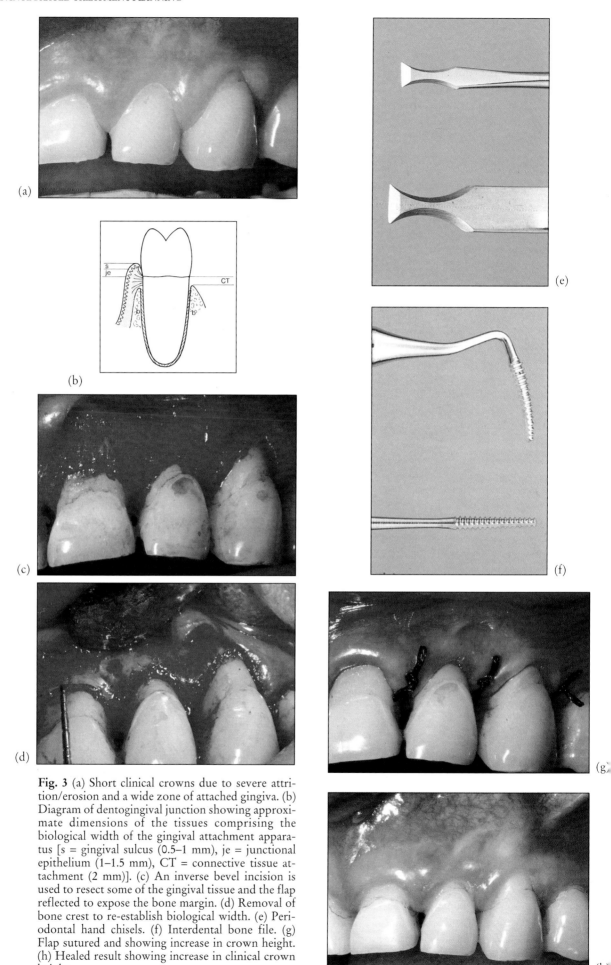

**Fig. 3** (a) Short clinical crowns due to severe attrition/erosion and a wide zone of attached gingiva. (b) Diagram of dentogingival junction showing approximate dimensions of the tissues comprising the biological width of the gingival attachment apparatus [s = gingival sulcus (0.5–1 mm), je = junctional epithelium (1–1.5 mm), CT = connective tissue attachment (2 mm)]. (c) An inverse bevel incision is used to resect some of the gingival tissue and the flap reflected to expose the bone margin. (d) Removal of bone crest to re-establish biological width. (e) Periodontal hand chisels. (f) Interdental bone file. (g) Flap sutured and showing increase in crown height. (h) Healed result showing increase in clinical crown height.

required. Limited widths of keratinised gingiva should be preserved by using a crevicular incision. Where there is no pocketing at the normal dentogingival junction, any increase in crown height will have to be achieved by apical positioning of the gingival margin following adequate bone removal.

These are very important decisions and should not be left until the surgical appointment. It is strongly recommended that study casts are evaluated to determine how much tooth reduction is proposed during the restorative treatment and how much increase in clinical crown height will be required to achieve this and provide a retentive preparation.

Following elevation of the flap the distance between the bone margin and the cement enamel junction can be assessed. In patients who have not lost any periodontal attachment this is about 2 mm and this exposed root surface has healthy collagen fibres inserted into cementum. With reference to the amount of extra clinical crown height required, alveolar bone has to be removed to a level which will allow a width of approximately 3 to 4 mm between the bone crest and the planned level of the gingival margin (fig. 3e). It is very important to minimise trauma to the bone and root surface. Thick bone should be thinned using rotating burs and plenty of saline coolant. The thinned bone adjacent to the root surface can be cleaved off using sharp hand chisels such as the Ochsenbein or TG0. On anterior teeth bone height should be preserved as much as possible interdentally to support aesthetic papillae. Where interdental bone has to be removed purpose designed files are very useful (fig. 3f).

The flap is then sutured to cover the alveolar bone. When the flap has been apically positioned a periodontal pack is required to maintain the flap position during early healing. It should be remembered that crown lengthening the palatal aspects of the maxillary teeth must rely entirely on resection as apical positioning is not possible.

RIDGE AUGMENTATION
Pontic areas can be treated by grafting with various synthetic materials or using soft tissue grafts, bone grafts and guided bone regeneration. This is most conveniently dealt with in the next section as the principles are identical.

## Osseointegrated implants

GUIDED BONE REGENERATION
The techniques of guided tissue regeneration originally devised to promote reformation of lost periodontal ligament using exclusionary membranes have achieved considerable success in bone regeneration in implant treatment (fig. 4). The technique relies on precisely the same principles, that is exclusion of unwanted cells

allowing preferential ingrowth of the tissue required. This goal may be more readily achievable when one considers that it requires regeneration of one tissue rather than several and it does not have the additional problem of the effects of plaque contamination of diseased root surfaces. Guided bone regeneration is used in basically two situations:

1. To promote bone growth at an edentulous site prior to the placement of an implant or bridge pontic thereby enhancing aesthetics by ridge augmentation.

2. To promote ingrowth of bone around an implant which has been placed into an area in the jaw where there is not sufficient bone volume to

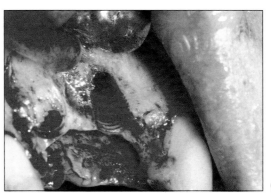
(a)

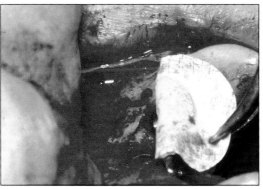
(b)

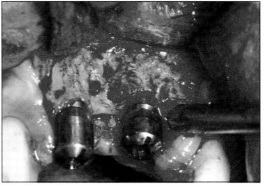
(c)

Fig. 4 (a) Implant site prepared at stage 1 surgery showing a deficiency in the labial bone. (b) The implant has been inserted and bone chips from an adjacent site placed over the deficiency and beneath a Gore-Tex membrane, which is secured with the cover screw. (c) Bone regeneration visible on removal of membrane 6 months later at stage 2 surgery (healing abutments have been connected to the implants).

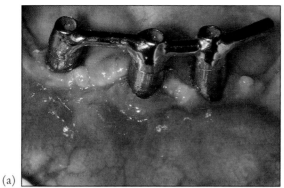

(a)

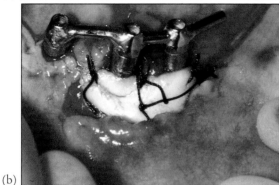

(b)

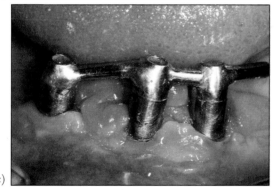

(c)

**Fig. 5** (a) Implant with no keratinised gingiva and inflammation of the alveolar mucosa. (b) Following surgical displacement of the alveolar mucosa, a free gingival graft is sutured in place. (c) Improvement in peri-implant soft tissues following a healing period of 6 months.

accommodate it. This results in either a marginal dehiscence or a fenestration.

The predictability of the technique is improved under the following circumstances:

1. The barrier membrane does not provoke an inflammatory response. Expanded PTFE membranes are very good in this respect.

2. The membrane is capable of maintaining a space into which the bone can grow. Materials are currently being developed which are stiffer and able to provide a greater degree of 'tenting'. Alternatively space is maintained under the membrane by using miniscrews as 'tent poles' or graft material such as autogenous bone (see chapter 5).

3. The membrane is stabilised against movement. This may be achieved with the cover screw if placed over an implant or with purpose designed mini-screws to secure the periphery.

4. The membrane remains completely buried under the soft tissues in a sterile environment with no communication with the oral cavity, ideally for several months. The results are compromised if membranes become exposed because the wound breaks down. This is a particular problem if dentures are worn over the site. It may be possible to keep the membrane clean using chlorhexidine but early removal of the membrane is advised.

5. There is sufficient bone surrounding the defect from several aspects.

6. Perforation of cortical bone by making bur holes may promote contribution from progenitor cells from within adjacent marrow spaces.

The technique has also been applied to the treatment of failing implants but that aspect is beyond the scope of this article.

SOFT TISSUE AUGMENTATION

Soft tissue augmentation using the equivalent of a free gingival graft (see chapter 6) can be used to provide attached gingiva around implants where mobile mucosa is readily traumatised and difficult to maintain in health by the patient (fig. 5). In situations where ridge augmentation is required simply to improve aesthetics, a subepithelial connective tissue graft is often the treatment of choice rather than augmenting the bony ridge.

# Conclusion

Periodontal management of patients is a key to the long term success of all treatment plans, but becomes particularly important in patients who are susceptible to periodontitis and those undergoing complex treatment plans. A guide to decision-making in treatment planning is provided on the following page. Techniques borrowed from periodontics can also facilitate management of some commonly encountered problems in other dental specialities.

# Decision-making in treatment planning

**1. Gather information**
Patient complaint
History complaint
Medical history
Clinical examination
Radiographs
Special tests

**2. Diagnose**

| Assess | Assess | Consider |
|---|---|---|
| Patient susceptibility | Prognosis | Treatment alternatives |
| — Periodontal | — Dentition | Treatment predictability |
| — Caries | — Individual | |
| — Other | teeth | |

**3. Discuss**

| Patient expectations | Treatment possibilities | Patient barriers |
|---|---|---|
| Aesthetic | | Psychological |
| Functional | | Physical |
| Dental | | Financial |

**4. Propose possible treatment outcomes**
*Definitive*: leading to a definite endpoint, eg a healthy, functional dentition with acceptable aesthetics or a complete denture
*Provisional*: leading to an intermediate stage in treatment to allow further consideration
*Compromise:** leading to a less than ideal endpoint because of unfavourable factors

➡

| **No** Reconsider plan | **Yes** Correct and proceed |
|---|---|

| **Not going to plan** Decide why Is it correctable? | **Going to plan — proceed** |
|---|---|

**Reassessment decisions**
following clinical and patient assessment

**Constant evaluation with formal reassessment at any stage in treatment schedule**
— *scheduled reassessment* at predetermined point in treatment plan
— *unscheduled reassessment* due to unpredicted event

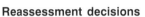

**Treatment scheduled and commenced**

**5. Decision time**
First ask:
Are you confident of the clinical assessment, prognosis and patient commitment?
Is it possible to define an end-point of treatment at this stage?
Has the patient been able to decide upon a treatment strategy from those available?
If *yes* to all of these questions proceed with definitive or compromise plan
If *no* to any of these questions proceed with provisional plan

**\*Factors leading to compromise**

| **Dental** | **Patient** | **Remember . . .** |
|---|---|---|
| Uncertain prognosis | Expectations | Your treatment planning decisions are usualy based upon the response of similarly treated patients. In addition it assumes the operator's familiarity and competence with the treatment techniques required. A specialist may be better equipped to carry out certain aspects of treatment and it may be advantageous to involve the specialist during treatment planning, especially in complex cases. |
| Poor root length/morphology | General health | |
| Distribution of remaining teeth | Age | |
| Aesthetics | Finances | |
| Inadequate bone for implants | Availability (eg travel) | |
| | Aesthetics | |
| *Unknowns:* success and predictability of other treatments necessary to the plan | *Unknowns:* motivation, compliance, tolerance, response to treatment | |

# 8 Management of acute conditions

This chapter covers:
1 Acute lateral periodontal abscess
2 Acute necrotising ulcerative gingivitis
3 Acute traumatic lesions
4 Acute herpetic gingivostomatitis

In comparison with chronic inflammatory periodontal disease, acute inflammatory conditions of the periodontium are relatively infrequent, but symptoms cause patients to seek help. The most common presenting acute condition is the acute lateral periodontal abscess. Acute conditions also include traumatic lesions, acute necrotising ulcerative gingivitis and acute herpetic gingivostomatitis. They display some or all of the classical signs of acute inflammation, swelling, erythema and pain.

## Acute lateral periodontal abscess

### Diagnosis

Acute inflammation with the accumulation of pus within a periodontal pocket and adjacent tissue produces a tender or painful swelling which tends to be relatively superficial (fig. 1). It is important to exclude the possibility of the abscess being due to an endodontic cause. There are a number of factors which help to differentiate the periodontal abscess (see panel top right).

The features listed below may be present in lateral periodontal and periapical abscesses and therefore do little to help in the differential diagnosis.

Features present in lateral periodontal and periapical abscesses
1 Tenderness to percussion (may be more severe in periapical abscess)
2 Increased mobility
3 Lymphadenopathy
4 Bone loss

Factors which differentiate the periodontal abscess
1 The tooth usually responds to vitality tests
2 There is associated pocketing on the affected tooth and on other teeth
3 In some cases multiple periodontal abscesses occur
4 An associated facial swelling does not normally occur
5 Pain is usually less than that encountered with a periapical abscess

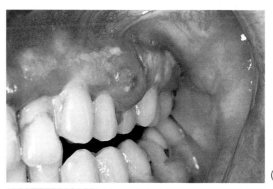 (a)

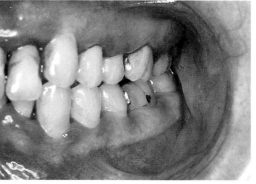 (b)

**Fig. 1** (a) A large, superficially located buccal swelling containing abundant pus. Deep pockets are present between the molar teeth, which are vital to pulp testing. Diagnosis: acute lateral periodontal abscess. (b) Resolution of the swelling following drainage and thorough cleaning of the root surfaces.

Evaluation of the pattern of radiographic bone loss may be helpful. Typical marginal horizontal and vertical bone loss are consistent with a periodontal cause, but an endodontic lesion from a lateral canal may also produce a similar pattern. Similarly, bone loss within a molar furcation could be due to either cause. An apical radiolucency may not be apparent in the early stages of an acute periapical abscess and in cases where the root apex is superficially located in relation to the labial cortical plate.

*Aetiology*

The aetiology of the acute periodontal abscess is multifactorial. Occasionally subgingival impaction of a foreign object or a fragment of calculus during scaling can be held responsible. It is often suggested that blockage of the drainage of a pocket may lead to the accumulation of pus. This may occur following resolution of marginal inflammation produced by oral hygiene and superficial scaling, but with failure to deal with more deep-seated inflammation. In patients where there are multiple periodontal abscesses it is more likely that this represents an acute imbalance between the host defences and the virulence of the subgingival microflora.

The host defence may be compromised, for example due to an associated viral illness or possibly fatigue and stress. A classic example is the impaired defence in patients with diabetes, and the possibility of an undiagnosed condition such as this should be considered in patients with recurrent/multiple abscesses. On the other hand there may be an imbalance in the microflora caused by overgrowth of a more virulent bacterial species.

Microbial shifts may occur within the complex microbial interactions in subgingival plaque, or consequent to alterations in the host, such as hormonal changes or the taking of antibiotics for an unrelated condition. Microbiological investigations of periodontal abscesses show mixed anaerobic infections with a wide variety of organisms, including the commonly encountered periodontal pathogens.

Key points in diagnosis and management of combined periodontal/endodontic lesions
1  Evaluate general periodontal condition and restorative status of involved tooth
2  Carefully probe entire circumference of tooth and examine furcations
3  Vitality test, preferably with both thermal and electric pulp testing
4  Take long cone parallel radiograph (with gutta percha point placed in pocket to help verify a communication)
5  Treat acute lesion — drain pus through pocket and/or root canal
6  Review — repeat examination and consider treatment alternatives
   a Extraction
   b Root canal treatment followed by periodontal treatment

*Management*

The acute inflammation and release of powerful enzymes from the leucocytes in pus may lead to rapid destruction of alveolar bone and periodontal attachment. This may represent the most destructive form of a 'burst' or exacerbation of the underlying chronic inflammatory lesion. If left untreated, the abscess will spontaneously discharge through the pocket or directly through the overlying tissue. The lesion will return to a more chronic state, but future exacerbations are likely. Simple treatment with antibiotics alone is not appropriate, as it will not affect the large mass of adherent subgingival plaque within the pocket.

The age-old maxim of draining the pus is the most logical and effective treatment, together with attempts to remove the cause. This is most readily accomplished by using a periodontal curette via the pocket entrance to drain the pus and remove subgingival plaque and calculus from the root surface. For the majority of patients this is a painful procedure and requires local anaesthesia, which can be given peripheral to the swelling or as a regional block. Use of an ultrasonic scaler will also help and provide good irrigation of the pocket. Some clinicians may also wish to irrigate the pocket with an antimicrobial such as chlorhexidine or a locally applied antibiotic. Adjunctive systemic antibiotics should be reserved for more severe cases, such as multiple abscesses and the presence of lymphadenopathy or pyrexia. The simple mechanical treatment should produce a rapid resolution of the condition (fig. 1b), resulting in shrinkage of the swelling and marginal tissue and prevention of further destruction of the periodontal attachment and bone. In cases where the tooth is considered untreatable, and particularly where there has been recurrent abscesses, extraction should be considered.

Following resolution of the acute phase the situation should be reassessed to determine whether the tooth requires further treatment such as root planing, periodontal surgery or extraction.

*Combined periodontal/endodontic lesions*

This is quite a complex subject, but can be readily dealt with by basic principles. In most cases periodontal and endodontic lesions are quite separate. For a tooth to have a combined lesion, the pulp should be non-vital and a communication should exist between a periodontal pocket and the pulp. Potential communications exist at the apex, and via lateral canals in furcation areas and the apical regions of the roots (fig. 2). There are many complex classifications of these lesions, but simply combined lesions arise when:

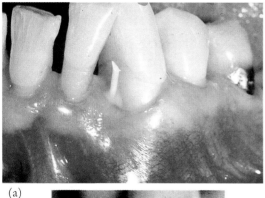

(a)

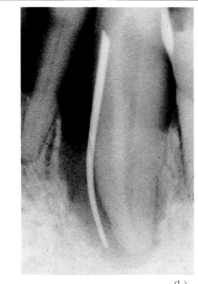

(b)

**Fig. 2** (a) Pus exuding from a deep pocket on the mesial aspect of a lower canine. A gutta percha point has been placed in the pocket to help clarify the extent of the lesion on radiographic examination. (b) A radiograph of the same tooth showing the gutta percha point extending close to the apex. In this particular case the tooth responded to vitality testing and therefore there was not a combined periodontal/endodontic lesion.

1. A periodontal pocket extends to involve the apex or lateral canal and this causes loss of pulp vitality. This is termed 'primary periodontal'.

2. A non-vital pulp causes an acute abscess which drains via the periodontal ligament. This initially forms a 'pseudo pocket ' which may be relatively narrow. This is termed 'primary endodontic'.

3. Both a periodontal pocket and endodontic lesion co-exist and progress to communicate with each other. This is termed 'true combined'.

In the primary periodontal lesions where the pocket has reached the apex of the tooth, the disease is very advanced and the tooth is often untreatable. Extraction of the tooth or affected molar root is indicated. Successful treatment of the primary endodontic lesion depends very much on how long the situation has existed. If the condition is diagnosed early and root canal therapy instituted the lesion may heal very rap-

idly. In this case there has been little chance of secondary plaque contamination of the 'pseudopocket'. Conversely, a longstanding lesion will develop the features of chronic periodontitis, and treatment will depend upon successful root canal treatment and periodontal root surface instrumentation. This type of lesion is much more difficult to diagnose and predictably treat. This is very similar to the case of the true combined lesion because it is not possible to determine to what extent each of the combined aetiologies has contributed to the lesion. In these cases it is recommended that the root canal treatment is carried out first, followed by periodontal treatment to cope with the residual pocket. All combined periodontal/endodontic cases are notoriously difficult to manage and predictability of successful treatment remains low.

## Acute necrotising ulcerative gingivitis (ANUG)

The incidence of this condition has declined over the last two decades but it is now reported more frequently in subjects who are HIV positive. Patients normally seek help because of pain which is constant and sometimes severe and because of increased gingival bleeding.

### Diagnosis

The affected gingivae are bright red and there is ulceration and necrosis of the gingival margin particularly affecting the interdental papillae (fig. 3). The ulcerated areas are usually covered

Most reliable diagnostic features of ANUG
1 Necrosis and ulceration of papillae
2 Pain
3 Bleeding

with a yellow/grey slough and are very tender to probe. Bleeding is readily elicited. There is often an associated lymphadenopathy, but pyrexia is unusual. Classically patients are said to complain of a metallic taste and there is a marked halitosis. In patients where the condition is severe, recurrent or becomes chronic there is usually destruction of bone and periodontal attachment (fig. 4) rendering the term 'gingivitis' a misnomer.

### Aetiology

ANUG is probably caused by opportunistic infection of the gingival tissue by commensal micro-organisms. It has been shown that spirochaetes invade the gingival tissue, and early studies suggested that a fusiform bacillus was also involved. Cultural studies suggest a more mixed anaerobic infection. The rapid resolution of the condition with the antimicrobial metronidazole supports the contention that spirochaetes/anaerobes are involved. There are, however a number of factors which predispose an individual to ANUG.

Smoking and stress may be linked in some individuals, and poorer standards of oral hygiene have been noted in smokers. In many reports practically all patients presenting with ANUG are smokers. The effect of smoking on

Factors predisposing to ANUG
1 Smoking
2 Stress
3 Fatigue and physical debilitation
4 HIV infection
5 Immunocompromised
6 Pre-existing gingival inflammation and plaque retentive factors

the vasculature and neutrophil function have been implicated in the aetiology.

### ANUG and HIV

Patients who are HIV positive, who may or may not be aware of their status, sometimes present with ANUG. It has been suggested by some clinicians that HIV infection should always be suspected in cases of ANUG. However, it is important to consider all the predisposing factors in an individual case, before suspecting HIV infection. HIV infection is more likely to be an aetiological factor in cases where there has been advanced destruction leading to exposure of alveolar bone. Persistent ANUG in these individuals leads to extensive destruction of the periodontal tissues. This type of lesion has been termed an HIV associated periodontitis or an ANUG periodontitis.

### Management

ANUG responds rapidly to systemic metronidazole 200 mg, three times daily for 3 to 5 days (fig. 3b). Penicillin and its derivatives provide a suitable alternative. However, recurrence is possible unless plaque control is instituted as soon as possible and any plaque retentive factors are removed by the clinician. It is therefore important to carry out a review and debridement within one week of the start of the antibiotics. It is also useful to recommend an effective anti-plaque mouthwash such as 0.2% chlorhexidine in the early management because patients find toothbrushing too painful.

In many cases the gingiva will repair and remodel so that more advanced treatment is not required (fig. 5). However, if there has been more advanced destruction, it may be necessary to carry out periodontal surgery to correct persistent gingival and periodontal deformities which compromise future maintenance. In its simplest from this would involve a reshaping of the gingiva using a gingivectomy procedure (see Chapter 4).

Deep interproximal craters in the molar regions may prove difficult to manage even using the most sophisticated regenerative procedures (see Chapter 6).

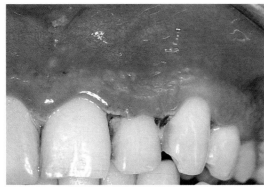

(a)

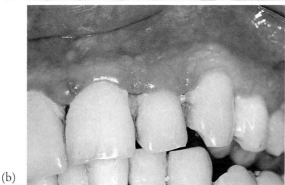

(b)

Fig. 3 (a) Ulceration and loss of interdental papillae in the upper incisor region. The tissues are very tender and tend to bleed spontaneously. (b) Resolution of the acute phase after a 5-day course of metronidazole. There is abundant plaque and the patient needs to improve their oral hygiene and have thorough scaling.

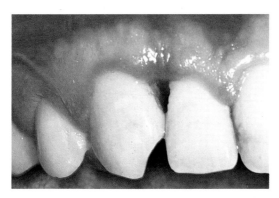

Fig. 4 Repeated attacks of ANUG have led to loss of papillae and a difficult aesthetic problem.

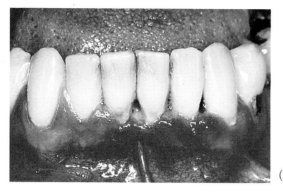

(a)

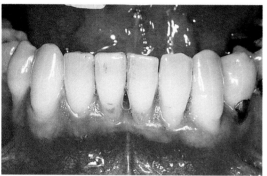

(b)

**Fig. 5** (a) ANUG affecting the lower incisor region. (b) Following a course of metronidazole and non-surgical periodontal care the tissues are healthy and have remodelled well.

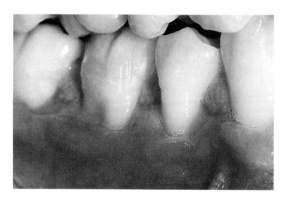

**Fig. 6** A persistent linear ulceration of the gingival tissue in the lower premolar/molar region. Note there is extensive recession but the interdental papillae are spared.

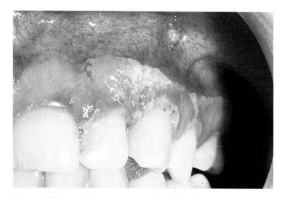

**Fig. 7** This patient presented with ulceration of the gingiva, palate and tongue. He felt unwell and had a pyrexia. Diagnosis: primary acute herpetic gingivostomatitis.

# Acute traumatic lesions

It is not uncommon for patients to damage the gingiva with toothbrushing. This may lead to a pattern of ulceration which generally spares the gingival margin and appears as a linear lesion across an interdental papilla (fig. 6). It is associated with an area of erythema and sometimes small adjacent patches of keratosis. Avid toothbrushing often results in gingival recession and cervical abrasion at associated sites. In patients who persistently traumatise the gingiva the ulceration can be extensive, of prolonged duration (sometimes several months) and the diagnosis not easy.

If traumatic ulceration is suspected the patient should be advised to stop all mechanical cleaning and use chlorhexidine mouthwash for a week. Traumatic lesions will resolve quickly providing the patient is compliant with these instructions.

# Acute herpetic gingivostomatitis

This condition is caused by the *Herpes simplex* virus and normally affects children and young adults. The viral condition produces 'flu-like' symptoms with pyrexia and lymphadenopathy. It is highly contagious and is spread from the lesions or secretions with an incubation period of about 7 days. In many patients the infection is subclinical, while in others they are more likely to attend their medical practitioner with the following signs and symptoms.

Signs and symptoms of acute
herpetic gingivostomatitis
1 Fever
2 Cervical lymphadenopathy
3 Stomatitis and pharyngitis
4 Oral ulceration
5 Gingivitis
6 Pain

The disease tends to be more severe in adults and the oral symptoms may make them seek the advice of their dental practitioner. The gingivae are bright red. Ulceration, which starts as small vesicles which rapidly burst, affects the gingivae and other oral mucous membranes (fig. 7). It should be relatively easy to differentiate from ANUG, although the two conditions have been reported to occur at the same time.

*Management*

Treatment is normally supportive by ensuring adequate fluid intake, analgesics, antipyretics and topical antiseptics. Antiviral drugs such as acyclovir are normally reserved for treating immunocompromised individuals.

*Reactivation*

The primary illness leads to infection of the trigeminal ganglion. Subsequent reactivation of the virus may occur. Most commonly, this manifests as herpes labialis which is often activated by sunlight. Intra-oral reactivation may occur following trauma such as surgery or even infiltration anaesthesia. It therefore occasionally occurs as a complication to periodontal surgery, particularly in the palate where it presents as a crop of small painful ulcers (fig. 8).

## Conclusion

Previous chapters have largely concentrated on periodontitis and gingivitis which are chronic inflammatory diseases, characterised by persistent bacterial challenge and the histological features of chronic inflammation. Periodontal abscesses and ANUG are usually superimposed acute conditions where the resident bacteria gain an advantage over the host defences. Both conditions are relatively easy to manage. Acute trauma may cause some confusion in diagnosis

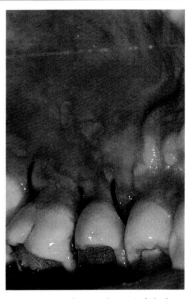

**Fig. 8** There is a crop of irregular painful ulcers on the palate, seen here one week after periodontal surgery. Diagnosis: reactivated herpetic ulceration

and herpes infection is not commonly encountered by the dental surgeon, other than as a reactivated lesion. It is important however, to recognise and manage all these lesions.

# 9 Osseointegrated implants in the periodontally susceptible patient

This chapter covers:
1 Basic guide to osseointegration
2 Teeth and implants
3 Periodontitis and peri-implantitis
4 Patient management

## Introduction

Osseointegrated implant systems which offer predictable long-term results backed by good scientific research and clinical trials are well established. They are an important advance and useful addition in the treatment planning and management of patients who have lost teeth or require extraction of teeth because of periodontitis. It is worthwhile reviewing the basic rules which govern the success of implants before considering the application in the usually more demanding case of the periodontally susceptible patient.

### Basic guide to osseointegration

Osseointegration has been defined as:
- A direct structural and functional connection between ordered, living bone and the surface of a load-carrying implant (Branemark 1985)

or more recently:
- A process whereby clinically asymptomatic rigid fixation of alloplastic materials is achieved, and maintained, in bone during functional loading (Zarb & Albrektsson 1990).

It has been proposed that the biological process leading to osseointegration is dependent upon a number of factors which include:

1. *Biocompatibility and implant design.* Implants made of commercially pure titanium have established a benchmark in osseointegration, against which few other materials compare. In addition, successful clinical results are reported for titanium alloys and hydroxyapatite coated implants. Screw shaped implants offer good initial stability at placement, a larger surface area and good load distribution characteristics. Some implant designs increase the surface area further by techniques such as 'shot blasting' or plasma spraying.

2. *Bone factors.* The most successful results are achieved in healthy 'good quality' bone. This is exemplified by a well formed cortex and densely trabeculated medullary spaces with a good blood supply. Examples of factors which compromise these features are infection, irradiation and heavy smoking. Success is highly dependent upon a surgical technique which avoids heating the bone. Slow drilling speeds, successive sharp drills and copious saline irrigation aim to keep the temperature below that at which bone tissue damage occurs (approx 47°C). The stability of the implant at the time of placement is very important. This is most readily achieved if the implant is placed so that it is engaged at both ends in cortical bone. This 'bicortical' stabilisation is not always necessary or possible, particularly due to anatomical limitations such as the presence of the inferior dental nerve. In general, implants placed in the anterior mandible have the highest success rate, as the available bone quantity and quality is more favourable than the maxilla.

3. *Loading conditions.* Following installation of an implant it is important that it is not loaded during the early healing phase as this would result in fibrous tissue encapsulation rather than osseointegration. To assist in this aim, implants may be countersunk to the bone crest and buried beneath the mucosa. Dentures should not be worn over the area for 1–2 weeks. In general, implants are left unloaded beneath the mucosa for approximately 6 months in the maxilla and 3 months in the mandible due to differences in bone quality. During this period the implant surface becomes osseointegrated with the sur-

Suggested minimum success criteria for dental implants (after Albrektsson and Zarb)

1  An individual, unattached implant is immobile when tested clinically.
2  Radiographic examination does not reveal any peri-implant radiolucency.
3  After the first year in function, radiographic vertical bone loss is less than 0.2 mm per annum.
4  The individual implant performance is characterised by an absence of signs and symptoms such as pain, infections, neuropathies, paraesthesia, or violation of the inferior dental canal.
5  As a minimum, the implant should fulfil the above criteria with a success rate of 85% at the end of a 5-year observation period and 80% at the end of a 10-year period.

ing of the implant-supported prosthesis is a further important consideration. Carefully planned functional occlusal loading will result in maintenance of osseointegration and possibly increased bone to implant contact. In contrast, excessive loading will lead to bone loss and failure (see below).

*Success criteria*

It is important to establish success criteria for implant systems, and for them to be tested in well controlled clinical trials. An example of the minimum success criteria proposed by Albrektsson and Zarb is set out in the panel.

Bone quality and quantity are very important factors governing success. Implants placed in the mandible (particularly anterior to the mental foramina) enjoy a higher success rate than the maxilla (approximately 95% success for implants in the mandible compared to 85–90% for the maxilla with systems such as Branemark). An example of the lowest recorded success rates are short implants (7 mm) used in the maxilla to support overdentures, especially when the implants are not joined together. A few studies have now demonstrated that the overall mean failure rate in smokers is approximately twice that in non-smokers. Smokers should be warned of this association and encouraged to quit the habit.

rounding bone. In partially dentate subjects, it is helpful and desirable to provide temporary/provisional prostheses, which are tooth supported to avoid early implant loading. This principle is illustrated in the case presentation at the end of this chapter. In some systems the implant is installed so that it protrudes through the overlying mucosa, and dentures have to be carefully relieved during the healing process to avoid premature loading of the implant. Following the osseointegration period the implant is exposed and components connected to it to allow construction of the prosthesis. The load-

# Teeth and implants

There are a number of fundamental factors to consider when comparing the biological and physical aspects of teeth and implants (left).

The gingival cuff around an implant abutment may be very well adapted but it lacks the fibrous connective tissue architecture of the normal dentogingival junction. The tooth is superbly adapted to differing functional demands because of the periodontal ligament. Excessive occlusal forces applied to the crown of a natural tooth will result in widening of the periodontal ligament, and an increased mobility. Under these circumstances the tooth is better adapted to cope with the increased forces. In contrast the osseointegrated implant is rigid within the bone, exhibiting no functional mobility. The attachment of the bone is such that successful adaptation is only possible by increased bone contact in response to carefully controlled forces. For example, the nature of the osseointegration does not allow orthodontic type movement of an implant and they have therefore been used successfully as orthodontic anchorage for tooth movement.

Excessive forces on an implant will result in either material fracture (of the superstructure, retaining screws, abutment screws or the im-

Healthy teeth versus healthy implants

| | *Healthy teeth* | *Healthy implants* |
|---|---|---|
| *Gingival junction* | | |
| Gingival sulcus depth | Shallow in health | Dependent upon abutment length and restoration margin |
| Junctional epithelium | On enamel | On titanium |
| Gingival fibres | Complex array inserted into cementum above crestal bone | No organised collagen fibre attachment — parallel fibres |
| Crest of bone | 1–2 mm apical to CEJ | At or about first thread in threaded implants |
| *Connective tissue attachment* | Well organised collagen fibre bundles inserted as Sharpey's fibres into alveolar bone and cementum | Bone growing into close contact with implant surface — oxide layer/bone proteoglycan and collagen |
| *Physical characteristics* | Physiological mobility due to viscoelastic properties of the ligament | Rigid connection to bone — as if ankylosed |
| *Adaptive characteristics* | Width of ligament can alter to allow more mobility with increased occlusal forces | No adaptive capacity to allow mobility. Orthodontic movement impossible. |

plant itself) or loss of bone contact to the implant surface. The latter may be evident as total loss of integration with loosening of the implant or loss of marginal bone. The latter type of bone loss is visualised as a radiographic saucerisation of the marginal bone and loss of bone contact along the implant surface. This has to be differentiated from bone loss due to bacterial-induced marginal inflammation or peri-implantitis, and once established may not be easy to determine.

## Periodontitis and peri-implantitis

The presence of periodontitis affecting remaining teeth or an individual's prior susceptibility to periodontitis may have an important bearing on success. Dentate individuals, particularly those with periodontal pockets, will harbour a complex microflora which is dependent upon an anaerobic environment and nutrient supply from the host tissues. It is quite possible that bacteria which are implicated in periodontitis, such as *Porphyromonas gingivalis*, are also the major pathogens in destructive inflammatory lesions around implants, the lesion of peri-implantitis. There is therefore a real possibility of colonisation or infection of the implant surfaces from pre-existing periodontopathic bacteria.

The destruction of the supporting tissues of teeth and implants have considerable similarities but there are important differences due to the nature of the supporting tissues (see above). This is particularly noticeable with the patterns of tissue destruction observed. Peri-implantitis affects the entire circumference of the implant resulting in a 'trough' of bone loss filled with inflammatory tissue extending to the bone surface.

In contrast, periodontitis-affected teeth commonly have irregular loss of supporting tissues, often confined to proximal surfaces and resulting in complex infrabony defects. In addition, for the most part the periodontal tissues are capable of 'walling off' the inflammatory lesion from the alveolar bone and periodontal ligament with a zone of fibrous tissue. It would seem probable that destructive inflammatory lesions affecting both teeth and implants have stages in which the disease process is more rapid (burst phenomenon) followed by periods of relative quiescence.

The incidence of peri-implantitis would appear to be uncommon, but can result in rapid destruction of the marginal bone which is impossible or very difficult to rectify even using modern regenerative techniques. Therefore, it is important that all patients treated with implants are managed in such a way as to avoid this complication, which may be more likely in the periodontally susceptible individual. This should be considered at all times in the treatment process:

1 Initial diagnosis and treatment planning.
2 Preparatory treatment including extractions, non-surgical and surgical periodontal treatment.
3 During the osseointegration period and any transitional stage.
4 Maintenance of the implant supported prosthesis.

The first two have been considered in detail in earlier chapters. This can best be illustrated in the form of a case study.

## Management of the patient with advanced periodontitis: the transitional case

A case is presented of a patient with advanced periodontitis, who had been treated 15 years previously with extensive bridgework in the upper jaw (fig. 1). This consisted of a telescopic reconstruction which was originally cemented to gold copings on the prepared abutment teeth (fig. 2). However, the superstructure had been uncemented for several years.

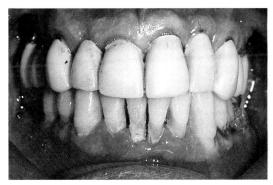

**Fig. 1** An anterior view showing a maxillary bridge extending from second premolar to second premolar. The gingival tissues are very inflamed and there are abundant plaque deposits. There is an advanced periodontitis affecting the upper and lower dentition.

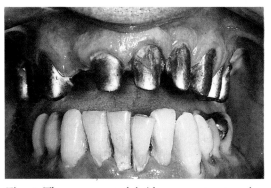

**Fig. 2** The uncemented bridge superstructure has been removed to reveal the gold copings on the abutment teeth.

Examination of the individual abutment teeth revealed excessive mobility (over grade 3), very deep pockets and radiographic loss of bone to the root apices and beyond. A limited number of teeth were amenable to treatment, the 13, 11, 21, 23, in the upper jaw and the 45, 44, 43, 33, 34, 35 in the lower jaw. The remainder required extraction. The patient requested restoration of the dentition with fixed bridges without an intervening period of removable dentures. A provisional treatment plan to commence periodontal stabilisation and carry out more detailed evaluation proceeded as follows:

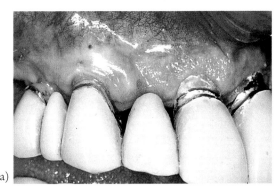

(a)

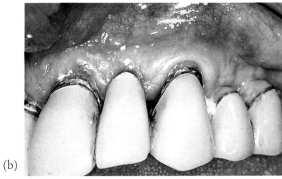

(b)

**Fig. 3** (a) right and (b) left views of the modified upper bridgework and the healed periodontal tissues following surgery. The teeth have a reduced periodontal support but the tissues are healthy.

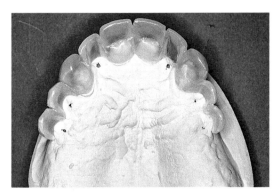

**Fig. 4** Surgical stent made to fit abutment teeth copings and providing labial faces of missing teeth to guide implant placement. Ideally, implants would have been placed additionally at the second premolar sites (marks on model), but there was insufficient quantity of bone to allow this.

*Provisional treatment plan*

1 Plaque control instruction and supra- and subgingival scaling.
2 Radiographic evaluation of the upper jaw.
   a. Long cone parallel radiographs of 13, 11, 21, 23 to check on suitability as interim abutment teeth.
   b. CT scan of maxillary bone to assess possibility of implant placement.
3 Evaluation of diagnostic casts and trial set-up.
4 Case discussion and definitive treatment planning. Plan agreed with patient to provide implant-supported upper bridge (using 13, 11, 21, 23 as interim abutments) and tooth-supported lower bridge.

*Definitive treatment plan*

1 Construction of an immediate replacement bridge for the lower jaw supported by 45, 44, 43, 33, 34, 35.
2 Modification of the existing upper bridgework to allow extraction of all teeth with the exception 13, 11, 21, 23.
3 Periodontal surgical treatment of remaining teeth to achieve:
   a. Pocket elimination and clinical crown lengthening.
   b. Establishment of a healthy dentogingival junction.
4 Modifications of upper bridge and re-preparation of abutment teeth (13, 11, 21, 23) to improve retention. This stage of treatment is illustrated in figure 3.
5 First stage implant surgery to place implant fixtures (Nobelpharma) at sites 14, 12, 22, 24 using a stent as guide for optimum placement (fig. 4). The upper bridge pontics to be modi-

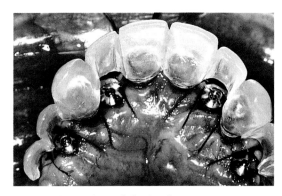

**Fig. 5** Mirror view of the implants at 14, 12, 22, 24 have been surgically exposed (stage 2 surgery) and healing abutments attached to them. The surgical stent has been placed on the abutment teeth to demonstrate the favourable position of the implants. The healing abutments are titanium cylinders which pass through the mucosa and protrude about 1 mm. The provisional bridge pontics usually need to be modified to allow recementation.

fied to allow recementation immediately after the surgery allowing for postoperative swelling.

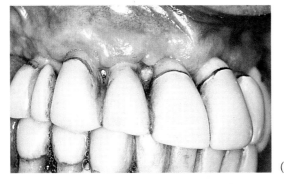

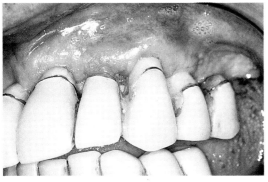

**Fig. 6** The bridge has been connected to the fixtures at 14, 12, 22, 24 via aestheticone abutments (Nobelpharma) and screw connection. At this stage the remaining upper teeth are removed and the provisional bridge modified accordingly.

6  Postoperative care and continuing periodontal maintenance.
7  Six months later to uncover implant fixtures placed at 14, 12, 22, 24 (fig. 5) and refit provisional bridge.
8  Modify bridge to allow connection to implant fixtures at 14, 12, 22, 24 (fig. 6) and extract remaining upper teeth. Provisional bridge now only supported by four fixtures.
9  Allow healing of soft tissue to cover extraction sockets (6–8 weeks) and place additional implants at 13 and 23 (unpredicted treatment required — new provisional bridge — fig. 7).
10  Allow 6 months integration period before exposing fixtures at 13 and 23 (fig. 8) and connecting healing abutments.
11  Final restorative phase to provide implant supported bridge based upon six fixtures at 14, 13, 12, 22, 23, 24 (figs 9 to 11) and definitive tooth supported bridge in lower jaw.

This is a complex and time consuming treatment plan with a number of advantages and disadvantages which should be appreciated.

*Advantages*

1  The patient is able to wear a fixed bridge throughout treatment, including during the immediate post-surgical phase(s).
2  It is particularly advantageous in those cases where guided bone regeneration techniques

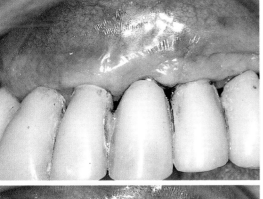

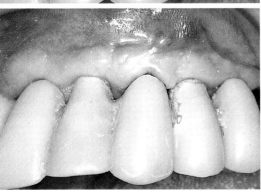

**Fig. 7** New provisional bridge connected to fixtures. The old provisional bridge had been modified to such an extent that breakage was inevitable and a new one had to be made. This was not predicted in the treatment plan.

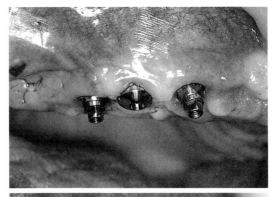

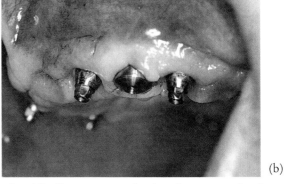

**Fig. 8** The fixtures at 13 and 23 have been exposed and healing abutments have been connected. The abutments on the fixtures at 14, 12, 22, 24 are aestheticone abutments (Nobelpharma) to provide screw retention to the provisional bridge.

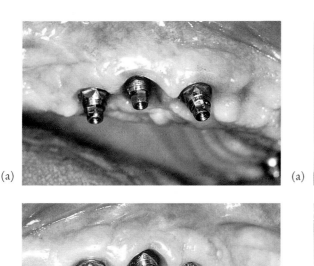

(a)

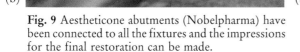

(b)

**Fig. 9** Aestheticone abutments (Nobelpharma) have been connected to all the fixtures and the impressions for the final restoration can be made.

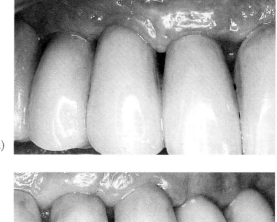

(a)

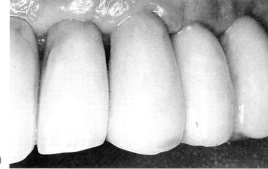

(b)

**Fig. 10** Fitting of the finished definitive bridgework. The crown margins are just subgingival and the embrasures are shaped to allow proper access for plaque control procedures.

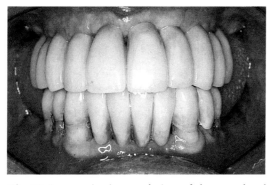

**Fig. 11** An anterior intraoral view of the completed upper implant-supported and lower tooth-supported bridges.

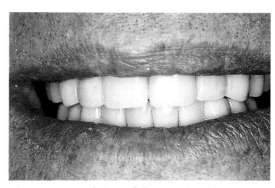

**Fig. 12** Extraoral view of the completed restoration.

with implanted membranes have been used because the overlying tissues are not subject to the forces and trauma of a mucosal-borne denture.

3 The implant fixtures can be progressively loaded.

4 Development and control of the occlusion is obtained at an early stage in treatment.

### Disadvantages

1 The planning is difficult and time consuming. It may be difficult for the patient to appreciate the large number of stages and the time involved.

2 The treatment is complex requiring a great deal of interplay between restorative and surgical disciplines:

### Restorative

It may be necessary to construct three to four bridges to satisfactorily complete the treatment. For example:

(i) Immediate insertion bridge with wire reinforcement and adaptation with resin to accommodate tooth extraction.

(ii) Provisional bridge with metal substructure and resin superstructure following periodontal treatment. This bridge is constructed to last over the complete treatment period until the final bridge is inserted. This could be over a time scale of 1 to 2 years.

(iii) An additional provisional bridge may be required to allow connection of the 'first wave' of implant fixtures.

(iv) The final bridge.

*Surgical*

Although it is sometimes possible to insert an adequate number of fixtures at one operation, it is often the case that there is not sufficient bone except where teeth are retained. The fixtures therefore have to be inserted in phases and bone augmentation techniques may be required.

3   Cost. The additional cost of the numerous bridges and extra surgical procedures is obvious. The additional time required removing and replacing provisional bridges on innumerable occasions is sometimes overlooked!

## Conclusion

The advent of predictable osseointegrated implants has provided a new dimension to treatment planning. In particular the treatment of the partially dentate and the transition from the terminal natural dentition to implant supported bridges provides a great challenge.

## Acknowledgement

Thanks to James Dewe Mathews for allowing us to show the restorative work in this case.

# 10 Patient communication of periodontal disease and treatment

The essence of good periodontal care lies in appropriate and adequate communication to the patient about the disease itself and the oral care required to maintain health. This topic deserves a chapter to itself because of the essential role the patient plays in initial treatment and long term maintenance.

Effective communication between the patient and the dental team is essential to good periodontal care. Improving a patient's understanding of their treatment and how they themselves can manage the health of their gums, will lead to greater satisfaction with treatment as well as improved compliance with dental advice. This guide has been written to help the dental team explain aspects of periodontal health, disease and treatment to the patient. The stimulus to produce this guide originated in postgraduate lecture courses given by the authors at which it has often been apparent that there has been a degree of uncertainty about how best to inform patients about periodontal disease and treatment. One of the most commonly asked questions was, 'What do you tell your patients?' This chapter begins by discussing some general guidelines for communication. This is followed by a summary of patient directed information relevant to periodontal disease and treatment.

## Guidelines for communication

Communication is a process of information transfer. In this particular setting the aim is to provide the patient with information on their periodontal condition and how this can be treated and managed. Effective communication depends on two broad factors — the characteristics of the message and the characteristics of the manner in which the message is presented.

### Characteristics of the message

The message should be clear and understandable. The clarity of message is aided if it has fewer conditional statements and is not likely to be contradicted by other information. While controversy may exist about some details of periodontal disease and treatment, the main points are established. In the following pages these main points are detailed both for the dental team and in a format suitable for patients. The ease with which a message is understood can be improved by avoiding the use of jargon and by using specific sentence structures. Sentences which are shorter and which contain fewer sub-clauses are easier to understand. What constitutes 'jargon' will depend upon the individual, however many of the specialised words and phrases used by the dental team may not be immediately understandable to patients.

General guidelines for communication
1 Avoid jargon
2 Keep sentences short and simple
3 Ensure that the message conveyed is consistent

### Characteristics of the manner in which the message is presented

The communication process follows a particular pattern as shown on the right. The process starts with the provision of information. This can be presented verbally, in a written format or in diagrams. There is good evidence to suggest that patients are more likely to remember information if it is presented in two forms simultaneously. For example, drawing a diagram while explaining to your patient the appearance of the tooth and gums is more helpful than describing

→ → Information provision
↑ ↓
↑ Frequent summaries
↑ ↓
↑ Clarification
↑ ↓
← ← Ensuring understanding

it in words alone. In providing information it is important to pay attention to the characteristics of the message — is it simple and is it clear?

Frequent summaries of the information which has been given so far serve as opportunities to recap and also as places to clarify any particular aspects about which the patient may be unclear. Allied to this is the attempt to ensure that the patient has understood the information presented. It is important that the dentist or other member of the dental team actively tests that the patient understands. It is not enough to assume that a patient has understood. It may be useful to ask the patient if they have any questions and to ask them to summarise any particularly important points. For instance, if a patient has been advised to use a mouthwash in a particular way — say holding it in the mouth for one minute — you may wish to ask them 'So can you just repeat for me how you should use the mouthwash'. Similarly the patient may be asked to perform a task — such as using inter-dental brushes — to demonstrate that they have understood the instructions.

When the clinician is satisfied that the information is fully understood they can provide further information if necessary. It is a matter of clinical judgement how much information the patient should be given. Individual patients will vary in the extent to which they seek information. In general most patients desire a certain basic level of knowledge and this is outlined in the patient information sections in this chapter.

The guide has been divided into the following sections:

> Guide to the disease
> 1 Healthy gingivae
> 2 Gingivitis
> 3 Periodontitis
> 4 Severe periodontitis
> 5 Gingival recession
>
> Guide to basic treatment
> 1 Oral hygiene and maintenance
> 2 Scaling and root planing
> 3 Periodontal surgery

The sections relating to 'guide to disease' are presented firstly in a patient directed format comprising clinical photographs, 'features box' and radiographs where appropriate. The sections relating to treatment are then presented in an integrated manner. This is followed by a series of line diagrams giving further information (at a basic and higher level) for members of the dental team (see pages 76–78). For certain patients a diagram through a tooth and periodontal structures can be helpful, together with relevant information at an appropriate level for the individual.

## Healthy gums

It is important for patients to appreciate the appearance of normal healthy gingivae, as this helps them identify health and disease in their own mouths. Some patients will prefer to look at a photograph of gingival health (fig. 1) while others may prefer to be shown healthy gingivae in their own mouth (providing this is possible). The features of health can be pointed out to them.

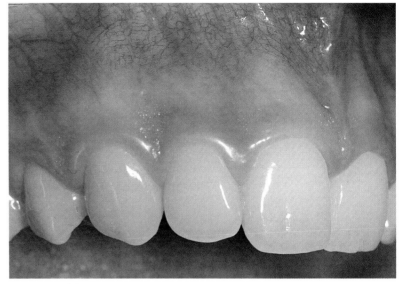

Fig. 1a Healthy gums.

Features of healthy gums
- Pink or pigmented, firm with a scalloped contour and no swelling
- Firmly attached to crown of tooth
- No bleeding on brushing or probing
- No plaque on the crowns of the teeth

## Gingivitis

When describing the features of gingival disease (fig. 2) the key points and features that should be mentioned are:
- gingivitis means 'inflamed gums' and can affect anyone
- caused by plaque at the dentogingival junction
- may develop in a few weeks
- can be treated with oral hygiene and scaling
- needs to be treated as it may be a precursor to periodontitis.

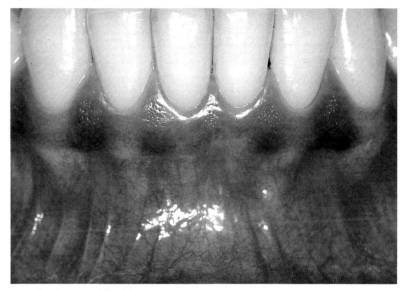

Fig. 1b Pigmented healthy gums.

Features of gingivitis
- Bleeding on brushing, eating or spontaneously
- Normally painless

When appropriate the features of severe gingival disease can also be mentioned.

Features of severe gingivitis
- Red, slightly swollen gingival margin (not entire width)
- Abundant white/cream coloured plaque adhering to tooth surface at the dentogingival junction
- Halitosis

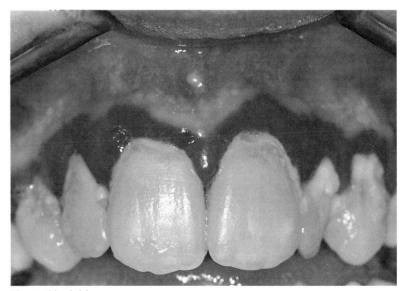

Fig. 2 Gingivitis.

## Periodontitis

When describing periodontitis the key points and features to make to patients include:

- the inflammation has destroyed periodontal support
- at first the teeth will be firm
- if left untreated will eventually lead to tooth loss
- x-rays reveal bone loss.

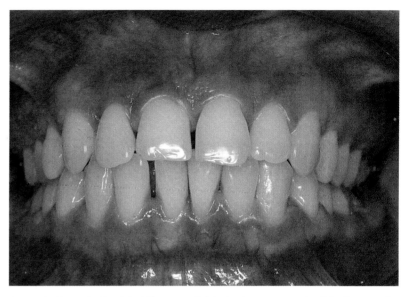

Features of early periodontitis
- Gingiva may appear almost normal
- Some teeth more affected than others
- Often painless
- Bleeding

**Fig. 3a** Early periodontitis. The superficial gingivae appears healthy but can be detached by 4–5 mm in many areas.

Figure 3 shows early periodontitis and can be used to illustrate how difficult it can be for the patient to understand the extent of the disease by just looking at their teeth in the mirror or waiting for any real pain or discomfort.

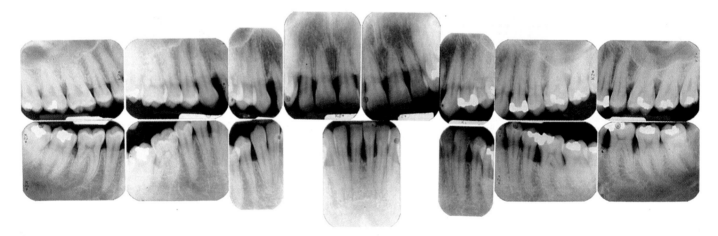

**Fig. 3b** Early periodontitis. The x-rays reveal the extent of the bone loss.

## Severe periodontitis

When the disease process becomes severe, the patient should be aware of:
- bleeding and mobility
- possible spacing between the teeth
- often still no pain other than sensitivity
- the possibility of abscesses.
- x-rays reveal that over half of the supporting bone has been destroyed.

Figure 4 shows severe periodontitis.

Features of severe periodontitis
- Bleeding
- Teeth may be mobile
- Spacing between teeth
- Abscesses

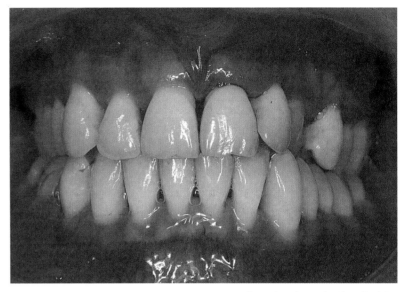

**Fig. 4a** Severe periodontitis. The gingivae are inflamed and can be detached by 7–8 mm. Bleeding occurs immediately on probing. The teeth are slightly mobile.

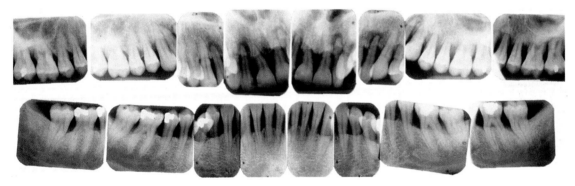

**Fig. 4b** Severe periodontitis. The x-rays reveal the extent of the bone destruction.

# Gingival recession

Gingival recession can often be a very difficult clinical symptom to treat, especially if caused by excessive brushing. These patients often feel a strong desire to 'keep their teeth clean' and do not feel happy applying less pressure. An explanation of the problem helps, but patients usually need more than a simple explanation to help them give up the habit of excessive brushing. Photographs such as those in Figures 5 and 6 can be helpful.

Figure 5a shows the mouth of a young individual with many areas of recession caused by excessive tooth brushing. This occurs most frequently where the pre-existing gingiva is thin, especially over prominent tooth surfaces such as the canine teeth (as shown). There is some inflammation of the gingiva because the brushing is incorrect, but there is no pocketing. This type of recession can be corrected by periodontal plastic surgery techniques.

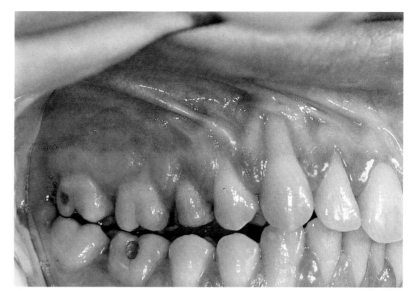

Fig. 5a

Figure 5b shows the same individual one year later following correction of tooth brushing technique and periodontal plastic surgery. This involved transplanting gingival tissue from the palate to cover the root surfaces. The gingival margin is now much more even and most of the exposed root surfaces have been covered. The gingivae appear healthy with no detachment and only small residual areas of exposed root.

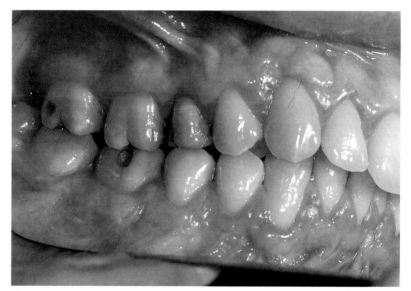

Fig. 5b

Figure 6 shows a large amount of gum recession resulting from periodontitis. The gum between the upper front teeth has shrunk to reveal the surface of the root. There has also been loss of the underlying supporting tissues including bone. This type of problem is not readily corrected by periodontal surgery.

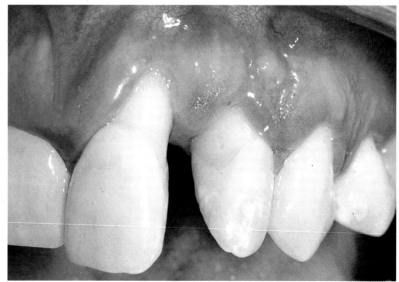

Fig. 6

# Oral hygiene and maintenance

The key to good periodontal health is plaque control. This aspect of treatment must be emphasised for patients in such a way that they not only understand the importance but also what they need to do in terms of basic oral hygiene. Some patients will want to know more about plaque and the disease process than others, so the information provided below should be tailored to the individual requirements and wishes of each patient.

## Plaque

The box below provides most of the basic facts about plaque that should help patients understand what is happening and why excellent plaque control is part of periodontal care.

> Facts about plaque
> - Plaque is the major cause of periodontal diseases
> - Plaque consists almost entirely of bacteria which normally inhabit the mouth
> - Plaque continually forms in all mouths and a visible film of plaque takes about 24 hours to grow
> - Plaque can be disclosed to make it easier to see
> - Plaque bacteria do not have to rely on food intake for their growth because adequate nutrients are present in the mouth especially when there is inflammation of the gingivae
> - The attachment of bacteria to the tooth surface is strong. The bacteria have to be dislodged from the surface by brushing, flossing and other oral hygiene aids
> - Plaque which is left undisturbed grows in thickness, number of bacteria and types of bacteria. It becomes potentially more harmful with time and can grow under the gingival margin
> - As plaque matures in this way some of the bacteria can produce an unpleasant odour, giving rise to halitosis
> - Some mouthwashes help to prevent plaque formation but they do not remove established plaque and they do not penetrate under the gingival margin
> - Plaque hardens or mineralises to form calculus above and beneath the gum

## Oral hygiene

Patients need good, clear and relevant advice on the correct method of brushing teeth and cleaning between them. They need to be reminded that the most critical area to clean is the gingival crevice, and that the bristles of the brush should be directed at this area and a small rotary or scrubbing action used to dislodge the plaque.

People who are susceptible to periodontal disease should be shown flossing techniques, and advised of the importance of interdental cleaning. The emphasis should be on results rather than prescriptive methods. People with larger interdental spaces will probably require devices such as wooden sticks and bottle brushes.

Patients may benefit from monitoring their oral hygiene using disclosing tablets. Use of photographs (fig. 7) beforehand may help them to know what to look for.

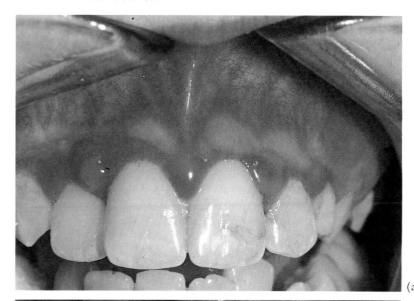

(a)

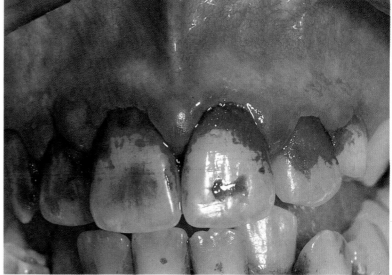

(b)

**Fig. 7** (a) This patient has inflammation of the gums and plaque growing at the tooth–gum junction. (b) The same patient after the plaque has been dyed with a disclosing solution. The plaque which has been present for over 24 hours is stained blue.

# Scaling and root planing

Many patients regard scaling of the teeth with pleasure but some regard it with suspicion. Thus where appropriate the dentist or hygienist should explain what scaling is and why it is beneficial. Root planing will usually be regarded by the patient as prolonged or more extensive scaling and while some patients benefit from a detailed explanation, others will be happy to accept root planing as part of the overall treatment plan. The box (right) provides some guidance as to the information that will help patients understand scaling and root planing.

*What to expect after treatment*

For many patients the treatment itself is less worrying that what to expect afterwards. Some imagine they will have no after effects and then are extremely concerned if they suffer some soreness or pain. Others are very concerned they will have a severe reaction and are extremely relieved to be told this is unlikely and that the worst they may suffer is soreness. Patients should be advised that the gums will usually feel a little tender and the teeth more heat and cold sensitive. Figures 8 and 9 show what is likely to happen.

Understanding scaling and root planing

*Superficial cleaning — scaling and polishing*

This entails removal of the 'chalky tartar' particularly from behind the lower anterior teeth and removal of stain by polishing with rotating rubber cups or brushes. This latter treatment is mainly for cosmetic reasons.

*Deep cleaning — scaling beneath the gum margin and root planing*

This is a more difficult and time consuming procedure. Many patients may find it uncomfortable and prefer to have local anaesthesia. Depending on how much treatment is required, several appointments may be necessary to treat a few teeth at a time. A patient with generalised moderately advanced disease could require four to six appointments of 30–45 minutes.

The dentist/hygienist uses basically two types of instruments:
- Instruments designed for manual scaling
- Vibrating instruments — these are fine probes that vibrate at a high frequency (often ultrasonic) which are cooled with a fine spray of water.

The dentist may advise using an antiseptic mouth-wash immediately after this procedure.

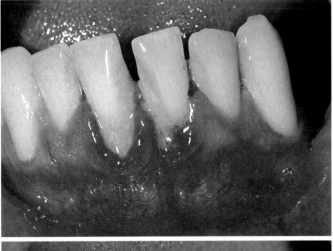

(a)

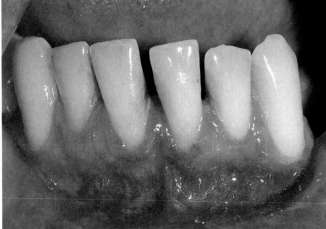

(b)

**Fig. 8** (a) Tartar growing near the gum on the lower front teeth. The gums are very inflamed because the tartar is covered with plaque. (b) The same area one week after the tartar was removed. The patient is not cleaning perfectly but the gums have improved in health and have shrunk back revealing the exposed root.

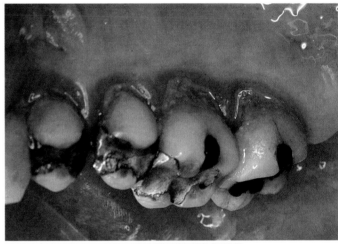

(a

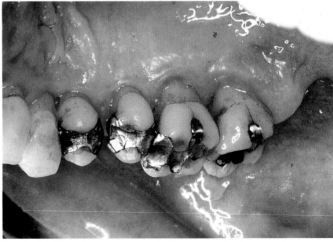

(b

**Fig. 9** (a) The inner aspect of the upper back teeth is an area commonly missed by patients. There is abundant plaque and tartar which extends beneath the gum margin. The gums are inflamed and receded. (b) The same area 6 months after removal of the tartar and improvement in the patient's cleaning. The gums are now much pinker, firmer and do not bleed. As the gums become healthier they usually shrink a little, exposing the root.

# Periodontal surgery

Although the word 'surgery' can be regarded as extremely worrying by a few patients, most appreciate honesty if the dentist suspects surgery will be indicated. Often the best way of describing it is to view surgery as an extension of scaling and root planing because the main aim of the procedure is precisely the same — the removal of bacteria from under the gingivae.

Surgery has the advantage of allowing direct access, inspection and cleaning of the root surfaces. It is usually performed to treat areas of more advanced disease which are persistent even after scaling and root planing (in patients who have proved to be capable of maintaining a high standard of cleaning).

The box here illustrates an example of the kind of comment that can be made to patients to describe surgery in an honest and accurate way. Figures 10 to 12 illustrate the type of changes that may occur to the gingival form or architecture following periodontal treatment including surgery. It is important that patients are made aware of and understand the possible sequelae of surgical treatment.

Describing surgery to the patient
Most surgery is performed under local anaesthesia. After the gum and teeth have been made completely numb, an incision is made to allow the gum tissues to be lifted away from the teeth. The deeper inflamed parts of the gum tissue are removed and the root surfaces of the tooth are thoroughly cleaned with the same types of instruments as for scaling and root planing. Some adjustments may be made to the shape of the gum. The gums are replaced around the teeth with stitches and sometimes with a dressing or pack.

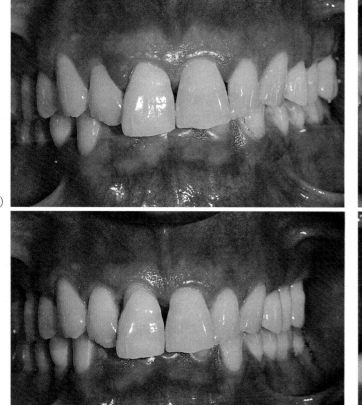

(a)

(b)

**Fig. 10** (a) The gum between the upper front teeth (arrow) is inflamed and swollen. (b) The same area after scaling, root planing and localised periodontal surgery. The margin of the gum is healthy and as a result there has been slight shrinkage of the gum exposing a small amount of root surface.

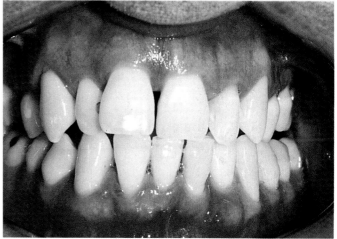

(a)

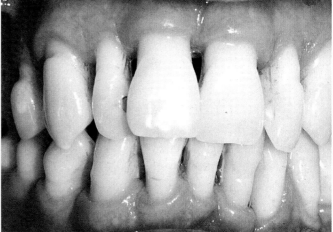

(b)

**Fig. 11** (a) This patient has generalised advanced periodontitis. The gum is very inflamed and detached with deep pockets and loss of about 50% of the bone supporting the teeth. (b) The same patient following extensive treatment including periodontal surgery. The gum margin is healthy but has receded by about 3 mm on all surfaces of the upper front teeth. The disease is now under control and the patient is able to clean the tooth–gum junction effectively.

Surgical aftercare

- The level of discomfort is variable and generally only requires painkillers such as paracetamol. It is better to take these before the local anaesthesia wears off and at prescribed intervals for the first 24 hours.
- It is not advisable to brush the area for the first week, therefore a mouthwash containing chlorhexidine is recommended to keep the area free of plaque. The mouthwash is held in the mouth for one minute and repeated twice daily.
- If any bleeding is experienced, locally applied pressure with a finger or damp gauze is usually sufficient to stop it. Complications such as bleeding or swelling are unusual.
- The stitches are removed after approximately 7 days and the healing reviewed by the dentist. Some gentle cleaning is carried out and advice given as to whether brushing can recommence or whether to continue with the mouthwash.
- You will need to be seen within a few weeks to monitor your progress and check that your cleaning is good. Your cleaning methods may have to be modified slightly. A number of visits may be needed during the healing period.
- There is usually some shrinkage of the gum margin immediately following surgery and as the tissues heal and mature. As a result the teeth may be more sensitive for a while.

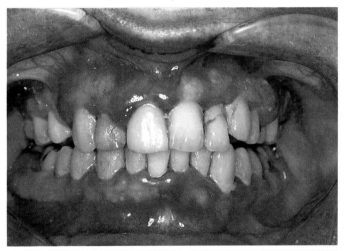

(a)

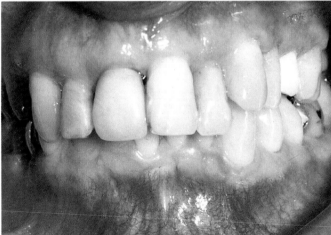

(b)

**Fig. 12** (a) A patient with generalised advanced periodontitis and many abscesses. These swellings are painful and are discharging pus. (b) The same patient after extensive periodontal treatment including surgery and routine regular maintenance care over a period of 15 years. The gums have been kept healthy by diligent cleaning by the patient and professional care. There is little shrinkage of the gum and the appearance is good.

*Aftercare*

A recommended explanation for surgical after-care appears on the left and may be more appropriate in written form as well as described by the dentist, nurse or hygienist.

*Long-term care*

Some authorities have demonstrated that the long term maintenance is the most important predictor of success in periodontal care. This must be explained very carefully to patients because there is a tendency for people to imagine that the end of a course of treatment means they are 'cured' of the disease and there is inevitably a tendency to relax on their oral hygiene regimen. The most important factor in maintaining gum health is the daily removal of plaque from the tooth–gum junction by the patient. Most patients find it necessary to see the dentist or hygienist at regular intervals.

## Conclusion

Patient communication is a very important part of periodontal therapy, often not appreciated or stressed in periodontal texts as much as it should be. Most members of the dental team receive little, if any, training in communication skills, and although a good communication technique is often common sense, there are certain guidelines that help.

Communicators need to remember that different patients will have different levels of understanding, different requirements and different levels of intelligence. If communicators ensure they always put the needs of the patient first and provide adequate information in a simple and understandable way then the periodontal health of patients will be sure to improve.

## Appendix

Line diagrams illustrating the gums in health, gingivitis and moderate and advanced periodontitis appear on pages 77 to 79.

## Acknowledgements

The authors would like to thank Tim Newton and Mike Grace for their help with this chapter.

## Healthy gums

Diagram of section through healthy tooth and periodontal structures showing the dentogingival junction

## Basic level information

Bone supporting the tooth.

Periodontal ligament. This is firmly attached at both ends by fibres which insert into the bone and into cementum covering the root surface.

In health the margin of the bone is about 2 mm from where the crown of the tooth meets the root.

The gingiva is firmly attached to the neck of the tooth and the underlying bone by fibres and cells which stick to the enamel surface of the crown.

The gingival margin is quite thin and there is a shallow groove (about 1–2 mm) between it and the crown.

Any plaque which grows on the tooth surface should be removed at least daily.

## Higher level information

Radiographically it is often seen as a more dense lamina dura at wall of socket. The crestal bone margin should be well defined.

The ligament is approximately 0.1 mm in width. It is an adaptable viscoelastic supporting system that can increase in width in response to greater forces (thereby increasing the mobility of the tooth).

Radiographic examination, such as bitewings, confirm that the distance between the cement enamel junction and the bone crest is no more than 2 mm.

The epithelial attachment is formed by a hemi-desmosomal attachment of the junctional epithelium. Apical to this is the supracrestal connective tissue attachment, consisting of a complex array of collagen fibres. These constitute the 'biological width' between bone crest and gingival margin.

The gingival crevice is shallow (0.5 to 1 mm) but clinical probing records a greater depth due to the probe penetrating the junctional epithelium. This should not cause bleeding.

Early plaque colonisation is mediated by aerobic gram positive organisms that can adhere to the tooth surface.

77

# Gingivitis

Diagram of section through tooth and periodontal structures in gingivitis

## Basic level information

Bone supporting the tooth is unaffected at this stage.

Inflammation in the gingival margin is a defence response to the mass of bacteria in the plaque. Fluid from the blood vessels seeps out and provides a food source for the plaque.

The gingival crevice around the tooth is slightly deepened due to swelling. The gingiva is still attached to the enamel of the tooth.

Plaque forms continuously on the tooth surface and now extends slightly beneath the gingival margin.

## Advanced level information

Radiographically the cement enamel junction to bone crest distance should not exceed 2 mm, but there may be some loss of bone crest definition due to the proximity of the inflammation.

The appearance and severity of the inflammation may be modified by such factors as the level of female sex hormones (increasing inflammation) and tobacco smoking (decreasing signs of inflammation but compromising defence mechanism).

The probing depth may be increased due to false pocketing or probe penetration into the tissue. Bleeding is readily elicited.

Plaque is complex with many interacting bacterial species including gram negative anaerobes and motile organisms.

# Periodontitis

Diagram of section through tooth and periodontal structures in moderate and severe periodontitis

Moderate
(left)

Severe
(right)

## Advanced level information

The bone is not normally directly involved in inflammation and therefore the patient does not experience pain. The inflammation causes bone resorption over an approximate radius of 2 to 3 mm from the plaque in the pocket. This may result in fairly even loss of bone (horizontal) or angular bone loss (vertical) where the original bone volume was large enough to accommodate the size of the inflammatory infiltrate.

Pockets of 4 to 6 mm are considered moderate and those of 7 mm or greater as deep. The pocket is lined with epithelium and at the base still maintains an attachment (junctional epithelium) to the tooth surface. The epithelial pocket lining is irregular and in places may be thin or ulcerated. The dense infiltrate of inflammatory cells includes all cells typical of chronic inflammation and this replaces the normal connective tissues.

The disease may progress in a gradual fashion or in relatively short bursts of activity. It should be appreciated that the disease can progress without the pockets necessarily becoming deeper. This occurs because recession of the gingival margin may keep pace with attachment loss once pockets have reached a certain depth.

The pocket environment is anaerobic and the inflammatory exudate provides rich nutrients for the bacteria. There is a well structured adherant plaque on the root surface (which often mineralises to form subgingival calculus) and a non-adherent phase within the pocket containing motile organisms and spirochaetes. These bacteria together with species such as *Porphyromonas gingivalis* and *Actinobacillus actinomycetemcomitans* are specifically implicated in the pathogenesis of periodontitis.

## Basic level information

Bone supporting the tooth is destroyed as a result of the inflammation. The left side shows early bone loss and the right side advanced bone loss.

The gingival margin is detached from the tooth forming a pocket. This increases in depth with increasing destruction of supporting tissue or swelling of the gingival margin.

Recession of the gingival margin often occurs as the disease progresses.

Plaque grows down the root surface into the pocket and causes inflammation of the tissues which is quite deep seated.

# Further reading

This reading list is mainly scientific
papers from peer-reviewed journals

## Aetiology and pathogenesis of periodontal disease

Genco R. Host responses in periodontal diseases: current concepts. *J Periodontol* 1992; **63**: 338–355.

Moore W E C, Moore L H, Ranney R R *et al* The microflora of periodontal sites showing active destructive progression. *J Clin Periodontol* 1991; **18**: 729–739.

Page R C. Gingivitis. *J Clin Periodontol* 1986; **13**: 345–355.

Page R C, Shroeder H E. Pathogenesis of inflammatory periodontal disease. A summary of current work. *Lab Invest* 1976; **33**: 235–249.

Seymour G J, Gemmell E, Reinhardt R A, Eastcott J, Taubman M A. Immunopathogenesis of chronic inflammatory periodontal disease: cellular and molecular mechanisms. *J Periodontol Res* 1993; **28**: 478–486.

Socransky S S, Haffajee A D. The bacterial etiology of destructive periodontal diseases: current concepts. *J Periodontol* 1992; **63**: 322–331.

## Chapter 1

Aucott D M, Ashley F P. Assessment of the WHO partial recording approach in identification of individuals highly susceptible to periodontitis. *Community Dent Oral Epidemiol* 1986; **14**: 152–155.

*Periodontology in general dental practice in the United Kingdom: a first policy statement*. Published by the British Society of Periodontology. Revised and reprinted 1994.

Buckley L A. An investigation of a simple method for screening periodontal patients in general practice. *J Ir Dent Assoc* 1988; **34**: 138–142.

Greenstein G. Advances in periodontal disease diagnosis. *Int J Periodont Restor Dent* 1990; **10**: 351–375.

Griffiths G S, Wilton J M A, Curtis M A *et al*. Detection of high-risk groups and individuals for periodontal diseases: clinical assessment of the periodontium. *J Clin Periodontol* 1988; **15**: 403–410.

Hausmann E. A contemporary perspective on techniques for the clinical assessment of alveolar bone. *J Periodontol* 1990; **61**: 149–156.

Lang N P, Nyman S, Senn C, Joss A. Bleeding on probing as it relates to probing pressure and gingival health. *J Clin Periodontol* 1991; **18**: 257–261.

Listgarten M A. Periodontal probing: what does it mean? *J Clin Periodontol* 1980; **7**: 165–176.

Loe H, Anerud A, Boysen H. The natural history of periodontal disease in man: prevalence, severity and extent of gingival recession. *J Periodontol* 1992; **63**: 489–495.

Osborn J, Stoltenberg J, Huso B, Aeppli D, Pihlstrom B. Comparison of measurement variability using standard and constant force probes. *J Periodontol* 1990; **61**: 497–503.

## Chapter 2

Becker W, Berg L, Becker B E. Untreated periodontal disease: a longitudinal study. *J Periodontol* 1979; **50**: 234–244.

Greenstein G, Caton J. Periodontal disease activity: a critical assessment. *J Periodontol* 1990; **61**: 543–552.

Jeffcoat M K, Reddy M S. Progression of probing attachment loss in adult periodontitis. *J Periodontol* 1991; **62**: 185–189.

Jeffcoat M. Radiographic methods for detection of progressive alveolar bone loss. *J Periodontol* 1992; **63**: 367–372.

Lang N P, Bragger U. Periodontal diagnosis in the 1990s. *J Clin Periodontol* 1991; **18**: 370–379.

Page R C. Host response tests for diagnosing periodontal diseases. *J Periodontol* 1992; **63**: 356–366.

Palmer R M. Tobacco smoking and oral health. *Br Dent J* 1988; **164**: 258–260.

Socransky S S, Haffajee A D, Goodson J M, Lindhe J. New concepts of destructive periodontal disease. *J Periodontol* 1984; **11**: 21–32.

## Chapter 3

Addy M. Chlorhexidine compared with other locally delivered antimicrobials. A short review. *J Clin Periodontol* 1986; **13**: 957–964.

Axelsson P, Lindhe J, Nystrom B. On the prevention of caries and periodontal disease. Results of a 15 year longitudinal study in adults. *J Clin Periodontol* 1991; **18**: 182–189.

Badersten A, Nilveus R, Egelberg J. Effect of non-surgical periodontal therapy. I moderately advanced periodontitis. *J Clin Periodontol* 1981; **8**: 57–72.

Badersten A, Nilveus R, Egelberg J. Effect of non-surgical periodontal therapy. II severely advanced periodontitis. *J Clin Periodontol* 1984; **11**: 63–76.

Caton J, Proye M, Polson A. Maintenance of healed periodontal pockets after a single episode of root planing. *J Periodontol* 1982; **53**: 420–424.

Corbet E F, Vaughn A J, Kieser J B. The periodontally-involved root surface. *J Clin Periodontol* 1993; **20**: 402–410.

Eaton K A, Kieser J B, Davies R M. The removal of root surface deposits. *J Clin Periodontol* 1985; **12**: 141–152.

Genco R J. Using antimicrobial agents to manage periodontal diseases. *J Am Dent Assoc* 1991; **122**: 31–38.

Greenstein G. Periodontal response to mechanical non-surgical therapy: a review. *J Periodontol* 1992; **63**: 118–130.

Greenstein G. Supragingival and subgingival irrigation: practical application in the treatment of periodontal diseases. *Compendium Cont Dent Educ* 1992; **13**: 1098–1129.

Highfield J E, Powell R N. Effects of removal of posterior overhanging metallic margins of restorations upon periodontal tissues. *J Clin Periodontol* 1978; **5**: 169–181.

Jones W A, O'Leary T J. The effectiveness of root planing in removing bacterial endotoxin from the roots of periodontally involved teeth. *J Periodontol* 1978; **49**: 337–342.

Lang N P, Adler R, Joss A, Nyman S. Absence of bleeding on probing: an indicator of periodontal stability. *J Clin Periodontol* 1990; **17**: 714–721.

Lindhe J, Nyman S. Long-term maintenance of patients treated for advanced periodontal disease. *J Clin Periodontol* 1984; **11**: 504–514.

Pallasch T J, Slots J. Antibiotic prophylaxis and the medically compromised patient. *Periodontology 2000* 1996; **10**: 107–138.

Paquette O E, Levin M P. The sharpening of scaling instruments: 1 An examination of the principles. *J Periodontol* 1977; **48**: 163–168.

Preber H, Linder L, Bergstrom J. Periodontal healing and periopathogenic microflora in smokers and non-smokers. *J Clin Periodontol* 1995; **22**: 946–952.

Rabbani G M, Ash M M, Caffesse R G. The effectiveness of subgingival scaling and root planing in calculus removal. *J Periodontol* 1981; **52**: 119–123.

Slots J, Rams T E. Antibiotics in periodontal therapy: advantages and disadvantages. *J Clin Periodontol* 1990; **17**: 479–493.

Tagge D L, O'Leary T J, El-Kafrawy A H. The clinical and histological response of periodontal pockets to root planing and oral hygiene. *J Periodontol* 1975; **46**: 527–533.

Torfason T, Kiger R, Selvig K A, Egelberg J. Clinical improvement of gingival conditions following ultrasonic versus hand instrumentation of periodontal pockets. *J Clin Periodontol* 1979; **6**: 165–176.

Waerhaug J. Healing of the dento-epithelial junction following subgingival plaque control. *J Periodontol* 1978; **49**: 119–134.

Westfelt E, Nyman S, Socransky S S, Lindhe J. Significance of frequency of professional tooth cleaning for healing following periodontal surgery. *J Clin Periodontol* 1983; **10**: 148–156.

Wilson T G, Hale S, Temple R. The results of efforts to improve compliance with supportive periodontal treatment in a private practice. *J Periodontol* 1993; **63**: 311–314.

# Chapter 4

Becker W, Becker B E, Ochsenbein C *et al*. A longitudinal study comparing scaling, osseous surgery and modified Widman procedures. Results after one year. *J Periodontol* 1988; **59**: 351–365.

Caffesse R G, Sweeney P L, Smith B A. Scaling and root planing with and without periodontal flap surgery. *J Clin Periodontol* 1986; **13**: 205–210.

Friedman N. Mucogingival surgery. The apically repositioned flap. *J Periodontol* 1962; **33**: 328–340.

Hill R W, Ramfjord S P, Morrison E C *et al*. Four types of periodontal treatment compared over 2 years. *J Periodontol* 1981; **52**: 655–662.

Kahldahl W B, Kalkwarf K L, Patil K D, Molvar M P, Dyer J K. Long term evaluation of periodontal therapy: 1. Response to four therapeutic modalities. *J Periodontol* 1996; **67**: 93–102.

Kieser J B. An approach to periodontal pocket elimination. *Br J Oral Surg* 1974; **12**: 177–195.

Lindhe S, Nyman S. The effect of plaque control and surgical pocket elimination on the establishment and maintenance of periodontal health. A longitudinal study of periodontal therapy in cases of advanced disease. *J Clin Periodontol* 1975; **2**: 67–79.

Lindhe J, Westfelt E, Nyman S *et al*. Healing following surgical/non-surgical treatment of periodontal disease: a clinical study. *J Clin Periodontol* 1982; **9**: 115–128.

Nyman S, Lindhe J, Rosling B. Periodontal surgery in plaque infected dentitions. *J Clin Periodontol* 1977; **4**: 240–249.

Nyman S, Rosling B, Lindhe J. Effect of professional tooth cleaning after periodontal surgery. *J Clin Periodontol* 1975; **2**: 80–86.

Ochsenbein C. A primer for osseous surgery. *Int J Periodont Restor Dent* 1986; **6**: 8–47.

Pihlstrom B L, McHugh R B, Oliphant T H, Ortiz-Campos C. Comparison of surgical and non-surgical treatment of periodontal disease. A review of current studies and additional results after 6 1/2 years following two methods of periodontal therapy. *J Clin Periodontol* 1983; **10**: 524–541.

Ramfjord S P, Nissle R R. The modified Widman flap. *J Periodontol* 1974; **45**: 601–607.

Rosling B, Nyman S, Lindhe J, Jern B. The healing potential of the periodontal tissues following different techniques of periodontal surgery in plaque free dentitions. *J Clin Periodontol* 1976; **3**: 233–255.

# Chapter 5

Bower R C. Furcation morphology relative to periodontal treatment. Furcation entrance architecture. *J Periodontol* 1979; **50**: 23–27.

Hamp S E, Nyman S, Lindhe J. Periodontal treatment of multirooted teeth. Results after 5 years. *J Clin Periodontol* 1975; **2**: 126–135.

Hirschfeld L, Wasserman B. A long-term survey of tooth loss in 600 treated periodontal patients. *J Periodontol* 1978; **49**: 225–237.

Muller H P, Eger T, Lange D E. Management of furcation involved teeth. A retrospective analysis. *J Clin Periodontol* 1995; **22**: 911–917.

Ross I F, Thompson R H. A long-term study of root retention in the treatment of maxillary molars with furcation involvement. *J Periodontol* 1978; **49**: 238–244.

Waerhaug J. The furcation problem. Etiology, pathogenesis, diagnosis, therapy and prognosis. *J Clin Periodontol* 1980; **7**: 73–95.

## Chapter 6

Becker W, Becker B E, Berg L, Prichard J, Cafesse R, Rosenberg E. New attachment after treatment with root isolation procedures: report for treated class III and class II furcations and vertical osseous defects. *Int J Periodont Restor Dent* 1988; **8**: 8–23.

Bernimoulin J P, Luscher B, Muhlemann H R. Coronally repositioned periodontal flap. *J Clin Periodontol* 1975; **2**: 1–3.

Caton J, Nyman S. Histometric evaluation of periodontal surgery II. Connective tissue attachment levels after four regenerative procedures. *J Clin Periodontol* 1980; **7**: 224–231.

Cortellini P, Pini Prato G, Tonetti M. Periodontal regeneration of human infrabony defects: V Effect of oral hygiene on long term stability. *J Clin Periodontol* 1994; **21**: 606–610.

Gottlow J, Nyman S. Barrier membranes in the treatment of periodontal defects. *Curr Opin Periodontol* 1996; **3**: 140–148.

Gottlow J, Nyman S, Karring T, Lindhe J. New attachment formation as the result of controlled tissue regeneration. *J Clin Periodontol* 1984; **11**: 494–503.

Langer B, Calagna L J. The subepithelial connective tissue graft. A new approach to the enhancement of anterior cosmetics. *Int J Periodont Restor Dent* 1982; **2**: 23–33.

Maynard J G. Coronal positioning of a previously placed autogenous gingival graft. *J Periodontol* 1977; **48**: 151–155.

Miller P D. A classification of marginal tissue recession. *Int J Periodont Restor Dent* 1985; **5**: 9–13.

Pritlove Carson S, Palmer R M, Floyd P D. Evaluation of guided tissue regeneration in the treatment of paired periodontal defects. *Br Dent J* 1995; **179**: 388–394.

Ripamonti U, Reddi A H. Periodontal regeneration: potential role of bone morphogenetic proteins. *J Periodontol Res* 1994; **29**: 225–235.

Schallhorn R, McClain P. Long term assessment of combined osseous composite grafting, root conditioning and guided tissue regeneration. *Int J Periodont Restor Dent* 1993; **13**: 9–28.

Seibert J S. Reconstruction of deformed, partially edentulous ridges, using full thickness onlay grafts. Part I Technique and wound healing. *Compend Continuing Educ Dent* 1983; **4**: 437–453.

Sullivan H C, Atkins J H. Free autogenous gingival grafts. I Principles of successful grafting. *Periodontics* 1968; **6**: 130–136.

Sullivan H C, Atkins J H. Free autogenous gingival grafts. II Utilisation of grafts in the treatment of gingival recession. *Periodontics* 1968; **6**: 152–158.

## Chapter 7

Garguilo A W, Wentz F M, Orban B. Dimensions of the dento-gingival junction in humans. *J Periodontol* 1961; **32**: 261-267.

Lundgren D. Prosthetic reconstruction of dentitions seriously compromised by periodontal disease. *J Clin Periodontol* 1991; **18**: 390–395.

Maynard J G, Wilson R D. Physiological dimensions of the periodontium significant to the restorative dentist. *J Periodontol* 1979; **50**: 170–174.

Melsen B, Agerbaek N, Markenstam G. Intrusion of incisors in adult patients with marginal bone loss. *Am J Orthodont Dentofacial Orthopedics* 1989; **96**: 232–241.

Nyman S, Lindhe J. A longitudinal study of combined periodontal and prosthetic treatment of patients with advanced periodontal disease. *J Periodontol* 1979; **50**: 163–169.

Polson A M. The relative importance of plaque and occlusion in periodontal disease. *J Clin Periodontol* 1986; **13**: 923–927.

Williams S, Melsen B, Agerbaek N, Asboe V. The orthodontic treatment of malocclusion in patients with previous periodontal disease. *Br J Orthod* 1982; **9**: 178–184.

Wise M D. Stability of gingival crest after surgery and before anterior crown placement. *J Prosthet Dent* 1985; **53**: 20–23.

## Chapter 8

Bergenholtz G, Nyman S. Endodontic complications following periodontal and prosthetic treatment of patients with advanced periodontal disease. *J Periodontol* 1984; **55**: 63–68.

Genco R J, Loe H. The role of systemic conditions and disorders in periodontal disease. *Periodontology 2000* 1993; **3**: 98–116.

Johnson B D, Engel D. Acute necrotising ulcerative gingivitis. A review of diagnosis, etiology and treatment. *J Periodontol* 1986; **57**: 141–150.

Porter S R, Scully C. Orofacial manifestations in the primary immunodeficiency disorders. *Oral Surg Oral Med Oral Path* 1994; **78**: 4–13.

Robinson P G, Sheiham A, Challacombe S J, Zakrewska J M. The periodontal health of homosexual men with HIV infection: a controlled study. *Oral Diseases* 1996; **2**: 45–52.

Scully C. Orofacial herpes simplex virus infections: current concepts in the epidemiology, pathogenesis and treatment, and disorders in which the virus may be implicated. *Oral Surg Oral Med Oral Path* 1989; **68**: 701–710.

Winkler J R, Robertson P B. Periodontal disease associated with HIV-infection. *Oral Surg Oral Med Oral Path* 1992; **73**: 145–150.

## Chapter 9

Adell R, Eriksson B, Lekholm U, Branemark P I, Jemt T. A long term follow-up study of osseointegrated implants in the treatment of totally edentulous jaws. *Int J Oral Maxillofac Implants* 1990; **5**: 347–359.

Albrektsson T. A multicenter report on osseointegrated oral implants. *J Prosthet Dent* 1988; **60**: 75–84.

Albrektsson T, Sennerby L. State of the art in oral implants. *J Clin Periodontol* 1991; **18**: 474–481.

Albrektsson T, Zarb G, Worthington P, Eriksson A R. The long term efficacy of currently used dental implants. A review and proposed criteria for success. *Int J Oral Maxillofac Implants* 1986; **1**: 11–25.

Becker W, Becker B E. Guided tissue regeneration for implants placed into extraction sockets and for implant dehiscences: surgical techniques and case reports. *Int J Periodont Restor Dent* 1990; **10:** 377–391.

Becker W, Dahlin C, Becker B E, Lekholm U, van Steenberghe D, Higuchi K, Kultje C. The use of e-PTFE membranes for bone promotion around titanium implants placed into extraction sockets: a prospective multicenter study. *Int J Oral Maxillofac Implants* 1994; **9:** 31–40.

Buser D, Weber H P, Bragger U, Balsiger C. Tissue integration of one-stage ITI implants: 3-year results of a longitudinal study with hollow cylinder and hollow screw implants. *Int J Oral Maxillofac Implants* 1991; **6:** 405–412.

Gunne J, Astrand P, Ahlen K, Borg K, Olsson M. Implants in partially edentulous patients. A longitudinal study of bridges supported by both implants and natural teeth. *Clin Oral Implants Res* 1992; **3:** 49–56.

Lindhe J, Berglundh T, Ericsson I, Liljenberg B, Marinello C. Experimental breakdown of peri-implant and periodontal tissues. A study in the beagle dog. *Clin Oral Implants Res* 1992; **3:** 9–16.

Nevins M, Langer B. The successful use of osseointegrated implants for the treatment of the recalcitrant periodontal patient. *J Periodontol* 1995; **66:** 150–157.

Palmer R M, Smith B J, Palmer P J, Floyd P D. A prospective study of Astra single tooth implants. *Clin Oral Implants Res* 1997; **8:** in press.

Palmer R M, Floyd P D, Palmer P J, Smith B J, Albrektsson T. Healing of implant dehiscence defects with and without e-PTFE membranes: a controlled clinical and histological study. *Clin Oral Implants Res* 1994; **5:** 98–104.

Rangert B, Jemt T, Jorneus L. Forces and moments on Branemark implants. *Int J Oral Maxillofac Implants* 1989; **4:** 241–247.van Steenberghe D, Sullivan D, Listrom R *et al.* A retrospective multicenter evaluation of the survival rate of osseointegrated fixtures supporting fixed partial prostheses in the treatment of partial edentulism. *J Prosthet Dent* 1988; **61:** 217–223.

# Index